The Mystery of Yawning in Physiology and Disease

Frontiers of Neurology and Neuroscience

Vol. 28

Series Editor

J. Bogousslavsky Montreux

The Mystery of Yawning in Physiology and Disease

Volume Editor

O. Walusinski Brou

14 figures, 1 in color, and 5 tables, 2010

KARGER

Basel · Freiburg · Paris · London · New York · Bangalore · Bangkok · Shanghai · Singapore · Tokyo · Sydney

Dr. Olivier Walusinski
General Practice
28160 Brou (France)

Library of Congress Cataloging-in-Publication Data

The mystery of yawning in physiology and disease / volume editor, O.
Walusinski.
p. ; cm. -- (Frontiers of neurology and neuroscience, ISSN 1660-4431
; v. 28)
Includes bibliographical references and indexes.
ISBN 978-3-8055-9404-2 (hard cover : alk. paper)
1. Yawning. I. Walusinski, Olivier. II. Series: Frontiers of neurology
and neuroscience, v. 28. 1660-4431 ;
[DNLM: 1. Yawning--physiology. 2. Respiratory Physiological Phenomena.
W1 MO568C v.28 2010 / WF 102 M998 2010]
QP372.M97 2010
612.2'1--dc22
2010001269

Bibliographic Indices. This publication is listed in bibliographic services, including Current Contents® and Index Medicus.

Disclaimer. The statements, opinions and data contained in this publication are solely those of the individual authors and contributors and not of the publisher and the editor(s). The appearance of advertisements in the book is not a warranty, endorsement, or approval of the products or services advertised or of their effectiveness, quality or safety. The publisher and the editor(s) disclaim responsibility for any injury to persons or property resulting from any ideas, methods, instructions or products referred to in the content or advertisements.

Drug Dosage. The authors and the publisher have exerted every effort to ensure that drug selection and dosage set forth in this text are in accord with current recommendations and practice at the time of publication. However, in view of ongoing research, changes in government regulations, and the constant flow of information relating to drug therapy and drug reactions, the reader is urged to check the package insert for each drug for any change in indications and dosage and for added warnings and precautions. This is particularly important when the recommended agent is a new and/or infrequently employed drug.

www.karger.com
Printed in Switzerland on acid-free and non-aging paper (ISO 9706) by Reinhardt Druck, Basel
ISSN 1660–4431
ISBN 978–3–8055–9404–2
e-ISBN 978–3–8055–9405–9

Contents

List of Contributors

S. Aboudan
Department of Psychology
University of Florence
Via di San Salvi 12
Complesso di San Salvi
Padiglione 26
50135 Florence (Italy)

James R. Anderson
Department of Psychology
University of Stirling
Stirling FK9 4LA (Scotland)

Julien Bogousslavsky
Center for Brain and Nervous Disorders
Genolier Swiss Medical Network
1272 Glion/Montreux (Switzerland)

Matthew W. Campbell
Living Links Center
Yerkes National Primate Research Center
Emory University
Atlanta, GA 30072 (USA)

Gregory T. Collins
Department of Pharmacology
University of Michigan
1301 MSRB III
1150 W. Medical Center Dr.
Ann Arbor, MI 48109 (USA)

Frans B.M. de Waal
Living Links Center
Yerkes National Primate Research Center
Emory University
954 Gatewood Dr.
Atlanta, GA 30322 (USA)

José Ramón Eguibar
Laboratorio de Neurofisiología de la Conducta y Control Motor
Instituto de Fisiología
Benemérita Universidad Autónoma de Puebla
Apartado Postal 406
Puebla, Pue. 72000 (México)

A.C. Gallup
Department of Biological Sciences
Binghamton University
Binghamton, NY 13902 (USA)

Fiorenza Giganti
Department of Psychology
University of Florence
Via di San Salvi 12
Complesso di San Salvi
Padiglione 26
50135 Florence (Italy)

Adrian G. Guggisberg
Department of Clinical Neurosciences
University of Geneva
Avenue de Beau-Séjour 26
1211 Geneva 14 (Switzerland)

Christian W. Hess
Department of Neurology
Inselspital
University of Bern
3010 Bern (Switzerland)

Johannes Mathis
Department of Neurology
Inselspital
University of Bern
3010 Bern (Switzerland)

Ramachandran Meenakshisundaram
Madras Medical College &
Government General Hospital
Park Town
Chennai 600003 (India)

Alejandro Moyaho
Laboratorio de Ecología de la Conducta
Instituto de Fisiología
Benemérita Universidad Autónoma de
Puebla
Apartado Postal 406
Puebla, Pue. 72401 (México)

Arunachalam Muthusundari
Tirunelveli Medical College & Hospital
Tirunelveli 627011 (India)

Fatta B. Nahab
University of Miami Miller
School of Medicine
1120 NW 14th Street, Suite 1347 (C215)
Miami, FL 33136 (USA)

Steven M. Platek
Georgia Gwinnett College
Lawrenceville, GA 30043 (USA)

Piero Salzarulo
Department of Psychology
University of Florence
Via di San Salvi 12
Complesso di San Salvi
Padiglione 26
50135 Florence (Italy)

Atsushi Senju
Centre for Brain and Cognitive
Development
Birkbeck University of London
Malet Street
London WC1E 7HX (UK)

Wolter Seuntjens
J.-F. Leemanslaan 27
1160 Oudergem Brussels (Belgium)

Shah Sweni
University of Debrecen
Medical & Health Science Center
Nagyerdei krt. 98
PO Box 48
4032 Debrecen (Hungary)

PonniahThirumalaikolundusubramanian
Chennai Medical College Hospital &
Research Center
Irungalur, Trichy 621105 (India)

Jaime Valencia
Laboratorio de Ecología de la Conducta
Instituto de Fisiología
Benemérita Universidad Autónoma de
Puebla
Apartado Postal 406
Puebla, Pue. 72401 (México)

Olivier Walusinski
20 rue de Chartres
28160 Brou (France)

I. Zilli
Department of Psychology
University of Florence
Via di San Salvi 12
Complesso di San Salvi
Padiglione 26
50135 Florence (Italy)

Preface

Along with laughing, crying, and even coughing, yawning is a mysterious and fascinating physiological phenomenon that has been poorly addressed. These phenomena share a complex paroxysmal motor-respiratory interaction that is strongly influenced by emotional factors. For instance, while the layman commonly associates yawning with boring situations, it also typically evokes a feeling of pleasure, especially during a full yawn with tonic extension of the limbs. However, many aspects of yawning remain unknown, and it will surely come as a surprise to many of us to read in the following pages that yawning may also be considered a strong sexual signal!

Dr. Olivier Walusinski is to be congratulated for putting together the fascinating chapters of this book, centered around a topic on which most neurologists would struggle to write more than a single sentence. The phylogenetic and ontogenetic (with fetal yawning) aspects highlight an interesting perspective on biological and human development, while the occurrence and features of yawning in neurological diseases also constitute an area that has only been explored by a few investigators. Dr. Walusinski is not merely one of these investigators, but an encyclopedic expert on yawning and its associated manifestations, as well as its neurobiological correlates. Moreover, it should be recognized that he has accumulated this large body of knowledge in parallel to his daily work as a general practitioner over the last 30 years! Acquiring scientific peer-recognition is not an easy task for an 'outsider', and we must say that the current result is beyond any of our initial expectations. Unlike most other books focusing on a specific neurological behavior or condition, the present work opens surprising windows into the history of neurology, human and animal behavior, and even philosophy; thus, making perfect 'anti-yawn reading'!

Julien Bogousslavsky
Glion/Montreux

Foreword

It is an honor and a privilege for me to introduce the first textbook in English dedicated to *The Mystery of Yawning in Physiology and Disease*. It is interesting to note that 30 years ago, much of the information contained in this book did not exist. Since that time, there has been an increased awareness that yawning is indeed a very pertinent model for understanding a transitional behavior and its determinism in terms of neuroanatomy, neurophysiology, ontogenesis, phylogenesis and social cognition.

Yawning has fascinated and mystified humankind for ages. The bizarre and evanescent qualities of yawning have invited boundless speculation about its origin, meaning and purpose. The neurobiological underpinnings of yawning have become increasingly well understood and it is now possible to describe the brain mechanisms responsible for the expression of this behavior in detail. Modern neuroscience is still looking for a complete explanation of its intimate purpose. We propose a broad-based cultural, ethological, neurophysiological, neuroimaging and medical overview of the related concepts.

Yawning is a stereotyped and often repetitive motor act characterized by gaping of the mouth accompanied by a long inspiration, followed by a brief acme and a short expiration. It is not merely a simple opening of the mouth, but a complex coordinated movement bringing together a flexion followed by an extension of the neck, a wide dilatation of the laryngopharynx with strong stretching of the diaphragm and anti-gravity muscles. Highly stereotypical because no environmental input changes the sequence of movements, it is observed in cold-blooded and warm-blooded vertebrates – from reptiles with rudimentary 'archaic' brains to human primates – in water, air and land environments. The ethology, neurophysiology and neuropsychology literature associates yawning with wake/sleep rhythm fluctuations, eating and sexuality, where it externalizes a group of possible vigilance-stimulating mechanisms and attests to the central role of the hypothalamus in homeostasis.

The chapters in this book represent the best thinking on the role and function of yawning, and they address what has become central to most contemporary accounts – the link between arousal, sleep, vigilance, satiety, sexuality and social communication linked to emotion.

As Winston Churchill said: 'The farther back you can look, the farther forward you are likely to see.' In this way, the first chapter tells the story of the prolonged effort in

Western thought to define yawning and to interpret it scientifically. Interest in yawning has existed since the dawn of history. Some of the world's greatest thinkers and physicians, such Hippocrates, Descartes, Diderot, Boissier de Sauvages, Haller and others, have attempted to explain the physiological and psychological bases of yawning. What is emphasized here for the benefit of the scientist or the practitioner is the evolution of the key concepts that define discoveries and developments in the field. For example, in his 1755 book *De perspiratione insensibili*, Johan de Gorter was the first to describe yawning as a mechanism to accelerate blood flow, supposedly to improve oxygenation of the brain, in response to cerebral anemia. Well into the 20th century, there were regular references to this notion, even though it had never been demonstrated. The inaccuracy of this hypothesis was formally shown by Provine, Tate and Geldmacher in 1987. In the chapter that follows, we shall continue to investigate popular thinking on yawning. We offer a broad-based cultural overview of the related conceptions and myths by comparing popular views in Arabic, Western and Indian cultures.

All the movements that a newborn is able to produce originate during fetal life and are performed throughout the life span. F. Giganti and P. Salzarulo explain that yawning is a behavior beginning in the first epochs of life. Their chapter examines frequency and time course changes of spontaneous yawning across the life span, taking into account hypotheses about its function and role. In recent years, there have been dramatic technical advances in diagnostic sonography. This procedure has become essential to the modern management of pregnancy. Fetal motility is considered to reflect the developing nervous system, but also involves functional and maturational properties of fetal hemodynamics and the fetal muscular system. Yawning is recognizable in ultrasound images from the 14th week of pregnancy, and like the appearance of oromandibular movements and swallowing, it signals functional maturation of the brainstem and basal ganglia. We hope to underscore the importance of fetal yawning with this chapter and depict how disturbances over time can lead to an earlier diagnosis of disharmonious brainstem maturation.

The relationship between spontaneous yawning and sleepiness is obvious. Sleepiness is a basic physiological need state linked to hunger or thirst, which are physiological need states essential to the survival of the individual. This implies a common functional basis, both physiological and biochemical, between sleep, arousal and yawning. Which structures and substances are implicated in the transition between waking and sleep and, at the same time, involved in yawning production? F. Giganti and P. Salzarulo review the relationship between yawning and sleep and highlight the contrast between morning and evening yawning. What can explain the fact that yawing, an expression of sleep pressure, can occur in its arousal time course (i.e. directly after sleep)? Further experimental studies can be considered after reading their chapter.

A. Guggisberg, J. Mathis and C. Hess also address this question in their chapter in which they review behavioral studies and electroencephalographic recordings of brain activity before and after yawning. The authors assess consistent evidence indicating that yawning occurs during states of low vigilance. For the authors, this substantiates the notion that yawning is provoked by sleepiness. However, studies analyzing autonomic nervous activity and EEG-based indices of vigilance in yawning subjects have not found specific autonomic activations or increased arousal levels after yawning. During sustained periods of taxing cognitive work, humans typically display time-on-task effects, in which performance gets steadily worse over the period of task engagement. Persistent effects of cognitive fatigue in the frontoparietal region after a period of heavy mental work indicate the critical role of this attentional network in mediating task effects. Can yawning be a marker of the level of fatigue in the neural attentional system by which a reverse attentional stimulation occurs, but not an arousal enhancement? Perhaps yawning is more a sign of some impending change of state rather than a statement of tiredness itself.

After completing his psychology studies, W. Seuntjens reviewed the scientific literature on yawning and found there was no simple and straightforward explanation of this phenomenon. He undertook his own research and wrote a thesis in 2004: 'On yawning or the hidden sexuality of the human yawn'. Here, he presents a summary of the data collected. Amassing circumstantial evidence, he substantiates the discovery of a hidden sexuality of the human yawn. Seuntjens uses the word 'chasmology', derived from the Greek, to describe the new field of research on yawning and foresees a bright future for it. Perhaps more philosophical than scientific, his chapter certainly appears to be the most original in this book.

Non-human primate yawns are usually categorized according to context (e.g. as a threat, anxious, rest or emotivity yawn), but there has been little consideration about whether these yawns are best regarded as a unitary behavior that only differs with respect to the context in which it is observed. James A. Anderson discusses the current view of yawning as non-verbal communication, whether champanzees can trigger voluntary yawns and how yawning by non human primates can be an opening into empathy. Reflecting the growing wave of research investigating these abilities, this chapter reviews the comparative literature and offers some thoughts relevant to the intriguing question: why does contagious yawning exist?

On the one hand, research on human stress has traditionally relied mostly on physiological and psychological measures with a relatively minor emphasis on the behavioral aspects of the phenomenon. A promising approach to the study of the behavioral correlates of stress is to analyze those behavior patterns that ethologists have named displacement activities. On the other hand, anxiety-related disorders are among the most common behavioral problems in humans and animals. On these occasions, animals frequently present lip licking, yawning or scratching, for example. In humans, yawning may even be a general preparation for some new mental experience. Certainly, people expecting something novel to happen indulge in yawning quite frequently; for example, parachutists about to jump tend to do so. Thus, yawning and stretching, like all forms of behavior, occur within definable contexts. Displacement activities are behavior patterns characterized by their apparent irrelevance to the situation in which they appear. Scratching, autogrooming and yawning are among the most commonly reported displacement activities in non-human primates, rodents, dogs and cats. Displacement behavior appears in situations characterized by social tension and is likely to reflect increased autonomic arousal. In such contexts, yawning gives more veridical information about the subject's emotional state than verbal or vocalized statements and facial expressions. We are proud to present new research, conducted by A. Moyaho and J. Valencia, in this promising field. Their work suggests that yawning is a delayed response to fear produced by response-dependent punishment in rats. The precise mechanisms whereby rats respond by yawning to emotional conditions remain to be elucidated, again suggesting a new field of investigations.

The past 30 years of research have led to a much greater understanding of the neuropharmacological regulation of yawning. While many of the early studies concluded that yawning was primarily driven by changes in cholinergic neurotransmission, Gregory T. Collins and Jose R. Eguibar expertly discuss the state of knowledge for each of the major neurotransmitters and neurohormones (dopamine, glutamate, serotonin, oxytocin, GABA and others) involved in the regulation of yawning, their interactions with one another, and their place in the hierarchical organization of yawning. This chapter is the most complete text ever published on the topic, and we predict it will be the most cited in the future.

A. Gallup has emerged as a leader in new perspectives on the function of yawning. His research provides support for the view that yawning is a behavioral response to transient hyperthermia, acting to counter intermittent increases in brain temperature and promote thermal homeostasis. Brain activity never stops. The brain is one of the most metabolically active tissues, generating large amounts of heat. Dissipating this heat as well as heat absorbed from the environment has been a major evolutionary hurdle necessary for continued brain development. It seems that the evolution of emissary veins (i.e. ritia mirabilia; the vascular network in the scalp and face removing heat from the brain) solved this problem. Brain cooling mechanisms have been described during fever to protect brain tissues and activities. There is no work (to my knowledge) indicating that cerebral activity modifies the internal temperature of the brain in a variable way according to the level of attention. Except during fever, the brain temperature remains constant; thus, how could yawning be necessary for brain cooling? This is the challenge that A. Gallup faces.

It has long been known that yawning is 'contagious'; ethologists speak of behavioral replication and neurologists refer to 'echokinesis', a term coined by J.-M. Charcot. The neural mechanisms responsible for spontaneous yawning as well as contagious yawning have been incompletely characterized. Fatta B. Nahab details how neuroimaging can be an essential tool for helping to identify the seminal neural structures and their inter-related functions to carry out this complex stereotyped motor program. Matthew W. Campbell and Frans B. M. de Waal point out that the various contagious yawning studies are confusing because researchers analyze their results differently. The authors go on to make recommendations for more rigorous, thorough and informative analyses. Their goal in raising awareness of these issues is to encourage new experiments and improve discussion of existing research. In particular, they propose more standardized studies of contagious yawning to test its hypothesized link to empathy.

Steven Platek summarizes the suggestion that contagious yawning is a primitive expression of social cognition, in particular empathy. Susceptibility to contagious yawning is correlated with speed in recognizing one's own face, theory of mind processing and is also associated with activation in regions of the brain that have been associated with social cognitive processes. This suggests that contagious yawning may be an evolutionarily old process that begat a higher level of social cognition in certain species. Atsushi Senju reviews the current evidence from developmental studies with typically and atypically developing populations and comparative studies in non-human animals. Developmental studies have revealed that contagious yawning is disturbed in individuals with autism spectrum disorders and schizophrenia, suggesting that contagious yawning may share a developmental basis with the capacity for theory of mind. He also presents comparative studies suggesting that contagious yawning can be observed in non-primate species and, perhaps, domestic dogs. His results seem consistent with the claim and previous statement that the mechanism underlying contagious yawning relates to the capacity for empathy.

As with all physiological behaviors, deregulated yawning reveals disorders. However, a property unique to yawning, which is nevertheless physiological, is its ability to trigger certain disorders and, conversely, to cure others! We successively cover all forms of yawning disorder – i.e. anhedonia, disappearance of yawning, excessive yawning – in a wide-ranging chapter.

The central nervous system in vertebrates follows a common organizational pattern and shows gradually increasing complexity with higher and higher levels of independence and functionality. A promising new field of research describes the pattern of associated movements observed in hemiplegic limbs during yawning. Thus, Ramachandran Meenakshisundaram and colleagues from India have collected 75 clinical cases of stroke. They indicate how, in certain stroke localizations, functional levels become disconnected; thus, functions may reappear that are normally inhibited by a phylogenetically more recent and functionally more sophisticated structure.

I would especially like to thank all my coauthors for their valuable work, which is essential to the success of this book. I would also like to extend a special thanks to Tanja Sebuk and Peter Roth at Karger for their active support and professionalism.

Dr. Olivier Walusinski, Brou

Walusinski O (ed): The Mystery of Yawning in Physiology and Disease.
Front Neurol Neurosci. Basel, Karger, 2010, vol 28, pp 1–21

Historical Perspectives

Olivier Walusinski

General Practice, Brou, France

Abstract

The phenomenon of yawning is just as intriguing and fascinating as sleep, yet understanding of its causes and consequences has defied the human mind for centuries. Hippocrates, Sennert, Boerhaave and de Gorter each advanced a theory in his time. From the release of tainted humor to the awakening of animal spirits and improved brain oxygenation, the metaphors that developed from these theories are all characterized by their popular success, which endured until the time of J.M. Charcot and even into our own day. However, starting in the early 19th century, a neuromuscular theory developed from the experimental physiology of Broussais and Flourens, which Dumpert (working in Germany after World War I) explained in detail. Experimental ethology and pharmacology in the 20th century brought the neuromediators and subcortical structures involved in yawning and pandiculation to light. Phylogenetically and ontogenetically primitive, these motor behaviors have been remarkably well preserved during evolution and are nearly universal in vertebrates. They are closer to an emotional stereotypy than to a reflex. Originating in the diencephalon, they appear to exteriorize homeostatic processes in the systems controlling arousal, hunger and sexuality.

Life, in all its aspects, has always given rise to thought and questioning. Explanations of physiological phenomena have always provided us with reassurance. As noted by H.L. Mencken [1]: 'Explanations exist and have always existed, because there is always a simple solution to each human problem, a clear solution that is plausible and false.' The history of knowledge on yawning is a perfect example of this precept. The causes and consequences of this intriguing phenomenon, as fascinating as sleep, have defied the human mind for centuries. The results of this review will inevitably highlight the numerous uncertainties that still exist in the 21st century.

Medicine originated in antiquity, from myth and philosophy, and gradually extracted itself from the uncertainties of magic and religion and moved towards a rational approach. This is illustrated in this chapter, which examines the development of our knowledge on yawning over several centuries.

In the tablets on Babylonian medicine that have been deciphered, there is no mention of yawning. Ethnomedicine, whether focused on Asia or Africa, has not studied yawning either.

Antiquity and the Middle Ages

Greek philosophy has provided us with a combination of 4 elements to explain the world (earth, air, fire, water). These elements carry the 4 physical qualities (moist, dry, hot, cold) that influence the 'humors' (black bile, phlegm, yellow bile, blood). These theories were applied in the first medical writings on yawning in *De flatibus liber*, a treatise on wind written by Hippocrates in 400 BC [2]. He observed:

> Yawning precedes a fever, because the large quantity of air that has accumulated ascends all at once, lifting with the action of a lever and opening the mouth; in this manner the air can exit with ease. Like the large quantities of steam that escape from cauldrons when water boils, the accumulated air in the body is violently expelled through the mouth when the body temperature rises.

As we will observe later, this idea persisted until the 17th century.

Discussing topics far removed from the physics he applied to humans, Hippocrates described jaw movement caused by yawning with great precision in *On the Articulations*, assimilating it into traumatic joint disorders. He related a reduction procedure incorrectly attributed to Nélaton in the 19th century [3]:

> With regard, then, to the matter on hand, the jaw bone is rarely dislocated, but is frequently slackened (partially displaced?) in gaping, in the same manner as many other derangements of muscles and tendons arise. Dislocation is particularly recognized by these symptoms: the lower jaw protrudes forward, there is displacement to the opposite side, the coronoid process appears more prominent than natural on the upper jaw, and the patient cannot shut his lower jaw but with difficulty. The mode of reduction which will apply in such cases is obvious: one person must secure the patient's head, and another, taking hold of the lower jaw with his fingers within and without at the chin, while the patient gapes as much as he can, first moves the lower jaw about for a time, pushing it to this side and that with the hand, and directing the patient himself to relax the jaw, to move it about, and yield as much as possible; then all of a sudden the operator must open the mouth, while he attends at the same time to three positions: for the lower jaw is to be moved from the place to which it is dislocated to its natural position; it is to be pushed backward, and along with these the jaws are to be brought together and kept shut. This is the method of reduction, and it cannot be performed in any other way.

Emile Littré [4], who translated Hippocrates' work in the middle of the 19th century, rendered a passage on the causes of apoplexy as follows:

> The continual yawning of apoplectics proves that air is the cause of apoplexy.

However, Jacques Jouanna refutes this interpretation in his recent translation:

> It is not obvious why paralyzed patients would be affected by continual yawning. There could be another explanation, namely that of patients constantly having their mouths open, which is observed in certain cases of paralysis [5]. The author, Hippocrates, has done his best to fit this observation into his explanation: the mouth stays open due to the continual presence of an excessive quantity of air in the body.

Nevertheless, modern medical observations indicate how right Littré seems to be!

Pliny the Elder noted in 40 BC that repeated yawning, when accompanied by extensive hemorrhaging, was a sign of approaching death [6]. This subject is the topic of a thesis in Latin, *De oscitatione in enixu*, written by Johannes Lapehn in 1758 under the direction of Johannes Roederer in Göttingen [7]. Hemorrhaging after delivery has killed thousands of women. The drop in blood pressure and the collapse triggered by hemorrhaging stimulates the autonomic nervous system. Yawning is an expression of this system, as it occurs during a vasovagal episode, and precedes loss of consciousness.

In his letter to Lucilius, Seneca wrote in approximately 50 AD [8]:

> Just as in weakened subjects, disease is signaled by precursory signs: either excessive nervousness, or a weariness unprovoked by effort; or yawning; or a shiver running through the limbs. In this way a fragile soul is struck long before illness befalls him, suffering by anticipation and succumbing ahead of time.

Is he talking about incubation, the onset of fever, somnolence or a depressive state?

Galen and Celsus alluded to Hippocrates by transposing the productive effect of yawning winds on the muscles. Following the line of Hippocrates' observations, Oribase wrote a chapter on causes and symptoms in 450 AD [9]. He lumped together convulsions, palpitations, hiccups, trismus, limb extension and yawning:

> They all belong to the same family, which involves perversion of muscular movements. […] Yawning and limb extension are acts of nature in which the body is forced to move violently by some kind of morbid cause.

In the 15th century, medical teaching began to change. Recitation of works by Hippocrates and Galen was replaced by descriptions of clinical cases and semiological ideas, spread through the invention of printing. *L'Universa Medicina* by Jean Fernel (1497–1558) is an example [10]. Fernel was the first to describe yawning as a prodrome of febrile states, calling it 'ephemeral fever'. Still influenced by the theory of humors, he described yawning as helping 'to evacuate harmful vapors'. In a similar vein, Jodocus Lommius published a collection of observations in 1560, *Medicinalium observationum libri tres*, printed in Anvers by Plantin. Translated into all European languages, this book gave rise to 30 editions over 250 years and can be compared to the modern-day *Merck Manual*. It describes yawning as a prodrome of fever [11, 12].

In 1624, Philippe Hechstetteri produced a similar collection of annotated medical observations (*Rararum Observationum Medicinalium)* [13]:

> Every day at four o'clock in the afternoon, a 14-year-old girl who had not yet started menstruating experienced very frequent, very irritating yawning followed by diverse morbific accidents.

He seems to be the first person, long before J.M. Charcot, to consider repeated yawning a sign of hysteria.

Scipion Dupleix, philosopher and historiographer of Henri IV and then Louis XIII, published a wonderful collection in 1626: *La curiosité naturelle rédigée en questions selon l'ordre alphabétique* (*Natural Curiosity Compiled into an Alphabetical List of Questions*) [14]. Not without evoking *Les Propos d'Alain* (by French philosopher

Emile Chartier), on the word 'yawn' he submits the following discussion to his curious reader, so well-phrased and close to our contemporary ideas:

> Why do we yawn when seeing others yawn? This is due to the common disposition of spirits or inside air, creating between us all considerable sympathy, consent and affinity, which moves and affects these spirits alike by recollection only. And for this same reason we cannot help singing when we hear others sing, our attention being otherwise occupied.

17th Century and the Birth of Research

The first half of the 17th century was marked by the birth of mathematical physics, creating a new vision of the world. A new scientific spirit was born with Descartes, resulting in the mechanistic paradigm in the field of physiology. After Galileo and Newton, the discoveries in mechanics and dynamics prepared the way for the concept of 'man as machine'. Until this period, medical dogmatism had led to a major error: an indifference towards research, as if medical knowledge were fixed and confined. After Harvey demonstrated blood circulation, the experimental approach opened the way to the quantitative analysis of vital phenomena, especially due to the work of Santorio.

Santorio Santorio (1561–1636), called Sanctorius of Padua, a physician in Venice and student and friend of Galileo, may be considered as one of the founders of experimental physiology [15, 16]. He tried to quantify physiological and pathological phenomena with measuring devices such as the scale, the thermometer and the metronome. With a scale of his own invention, he measured and compared weight gain and loss in humans, particularly by perspiration. He built an entire medical theory based on the weight differences related to nutrition, releases via the emunctories and perspiration, calling it static medicine. He mentioned yawning in his aphorisms:

> Yawning and limb extension after sleep show that the body perspires abundantly, similar to the rooster that flaps its wings before it starts to sing. The urge to yawn and stretch the limbs upon waking stems from the abundance of perspirable matter, creating an inclination to perspire. Through yawning and limb extension we perspire more in one half hour than we would during other times in three hours.

In 1664, René Descartes (1596–1650) exposed his theory on nerves in his 'Traité de L'Homme' ('Treatise of man'):

> The spirits that are in the brain enter into specific nerves; at the same time they carry the strength to move a specific limb. Having discussed respiration and other simple and ordinary movements of this type, I will explain how exterior objects act on the sensory organs.

Further on he explains respiration through the muscular activity of the diaphragm and focuses on 'how this machine swallows the meat at the back of its mouth …'. He concludes his complex explanation of aerodigestive tract functioning with the following:

> By way of example, you can also observe how this machine can sneeze, yawn, cough, and make the necessary movements to discharge a variety of other excrements.

This demonstrates that nearly 1,000 years after Hippocrates, the evacuation of humors was still considered a primordial effect of yawning [17].

Danieli Sennerti (1572–1637) also continued to assimilate sneezing and yawning as a mechanism of 'morbific exhalation', while pointing out the coincidence with fatigue and somnolence, which had never before been noted [18].

Jan Baptiste van Helmont (1577–1644) was the first to challenge Hippocrates' ideas in *Des principes de médecine et de physique pour la guérison des maladies* ('*Principles of Medicine and Physics for Healing Diseases*') in 1671 [19]:

> Galen states that the yawning usually accompanying the onset of intermittent fever is caused by sooty vapors that swell & distend the muscles of the jaw, from which they try to detach themselves. Why are these parts of the body more excited than other parts by expulsion of this sooty matter, given that the sooty matter can only be the imperceptible excrements of the most recent digestion? And why is this matter encountered more during fever than during gout, apoplexy, etc? Why do we yawn in spite of ourselves when someone else yawns? This demonstrates that yawning does not proceed from sooty vapors, but from the imagination. The school of medicine does not contest that the orifice of the stomach is easily moved & excited to nausea by disdain for something perceived or imagined to be dirty, & that when some people watch others eat sour apples, their mouths immediately fill with saliva. Thus the upper orifice of the stomach is easily moved by the imagination, and sleep, coma, bad mood, catalepsy, drowsiness, vertigo and other accidents of this type come from the orifice of the stomach. Yawning which follows or prefigures sleep is consequently attributed to the same part of the body, because phantasy resides there and it is not without reason that we call this place the heart. It follows that when we are noticeably afflicted, we sigh repeatedly which seems to relieve this upper orifice of its oppression. When the lethargic and nonchalant stomach makes us drowsy, taking the trouble to yawn does not give any release to the muscles of the mouth and trachea which are thereby engaged. Similarly, the ethmoid bone, disturbing the organ of smell, calls on the muscles of the chest for sternutation. This does not mean that the cause of yawning should be sought in the muscles that move when one yawns, no more than the cause of sneezing should be sought in the muscles that move when one sneezes.

Calling Hippocratic Theories into Question

Herman Boerhaave (1668–1738) is considered the founder of clinical medicine and the modern academic hospital. In 1680, in *Praelectiones academicae*, he provided the first novel explanation of yawning:

> Yawning and pandiculation favor the equitable distribution of spiritus in all the muscles and unblock the vessels of which sleep may have slowed the functions [20]. In certain cases, yawning and pandiculation favor blood flow and re-establish the nervous influx; their action fights the excessive predominance of the flexor muscles and returns everything to its place. [...] Yawning involves extending most of the muscles controlled by the will at almost the same time, while expanding the lungs amply and inhaling a great deal of air slowly and gradually. After the air has been held for some time and is rarefied, it is imperceptibly released by exhalation and the muscles finally return to their natural state. The effect of yawning is thus to move all the humors of the body through all the vessels, to accelerate their movement, to distribute them equally and as a result, to give the sensory organs and muscles of the body the capacity to perform their functions.

The dissertations of Johann Beutler (1685) and Gottlob Hermann (1720) build on these theories, adding a prognostic role to yawning, considered to indicate a fever's seriousness [21, 22].

Pierre Brisseau associated yawning and epilepsy for the first time in his *Traité des mouvements simpatiques* (*'Treatise on Sympathetic Movements'*) in 1692 [23]:

The signs of an imminent attack of epilepsy are a disturbance of the soul and the senses, heaviness and pain in the head, vertigo, irritating insomnia, weariness in the joints, trembling of the limbs, ringing in the ears, yawning, heart palpitation, difficulty breathing, nausea, cardialgia, etc. All of these signs are more or less present in epileptics. [...] Because blood circulates with difficulty around the lungs, yawning is easy to deduce in those about to be struck by a fit of epilepsy.

In 1733, George Cheyne (1671–1743) wrote *The English Malady: Treatise of Nervous Diseases of All Kinds* [24], in which he explains:

Yawning and pandiculation seem to be produced by hard concretions, by saline particles, by harmful vapors, bitter or acrimonious, by perspiration, by winds, etc., that are either in or stop in small vessels, or are carried to a part of the body with many nerves such as the alimentary canal, the cavities of the brain, the spine or the interstices of the muscles. Because the nerves in these places or their membranes are irritated, a general disturbance takes place in all nervous or sensible fiber, soon producing the same effect throughout the entire muscular system'. [...] 'Vapors, or splenic disorder, are commonly understood to refer to an excess of dejection, discouragement, bloating of the stomach, belching, noise in the lower abdomen, ringing or buzzing in the ears, yawning, lack of appetite, agitation, worry, anxiety, ill humor, melancholy, sadness, inconstancy, insomnia or drowsiness, or in a word all the symptoms that do not form a particular disease; but the vapors are very often symptomatic and depend on another malady.

The premises of J.M. Charcot's 'hystero-epilepsy' can be found here, and it was not until the 20th century that epilepsy, cortical pathology and hysteria, the psychological condition, were separated.

18th Century: Yawning 'Improves Brain Oxygenation'

Johannes de Gorter (1689–1762), a prolific Dutch author in all areas of medicine in the early 18th century, holds a key place in the history of knowledge on yawning. In his book *De Perspiratione insensibili* in 1755, he attributed yawning 'to a need for faster blood circulation and to cerebral anemia' [25]. This marks the birth of an idea that would persist for two centuries, repeated by almost all authors: yawning improves brain oxygenation.

Albrecht von Haller (1708–1777), a Swiss physician and poet, wrote the first compendium of human physiology (*Elementa physiologiae corporis humani*: 8 volumes published from 1757 to 1766). Following on from Francis Glisson, he introduced the notion of 'irritability', the property of tissues to be stimulated [26]. He was the first to record proof of this phenomenon and distinguished nerve impulses (sensitivity) from muscular contraction (irritability):

A kind of harmony exists between the pulse and the breath. In the natural state, there are usually three or four pulsations during one breath. If more blood reaches the heart, the number of pulsations and breaths increases. This explains why it is harder to breathe when the body is in motion, because the venous blood is whipped and accelerated. If there is greater distance in the lungs, and the blood has trouble passing from the right to the left ventricle, the number and length of breaths will be greater in order to cover the distance. This is the cause of sighs and yawning.

He goes on to describe sleep:

As night approaches, one feels a numbness in the long muscles and their tendons, together with an incapacity for serious thought and a love of rest. At this point, the forces holding up the body weaken, the eyes close, the lower jaw is left hanging, which forces one to yawn.

In the same vein as de Gorter, he advances the following:

Why do we yawn when we feel like sleeping? In order to clear the lungs in which the blood is moving more slowly.

David Hartley (1705–1757), an English physician influenced by the discoveries of Isaac Newton, attempted to explain human physiology using physical laws based on the laws of gravity. Like Hippocrates who transposed Aristotle's knowledge of nature into 4 humors, Hartley proposed that perceived sensations and voluntary acts were dependent on the vibration of particles that composed human tissue and were invisible to the eye, travelling the length of the nerves and thereby giving substance to the 'animal spirits' of Descartes. He therefore prefigured the concept of molecules [27–29]:

Depending on the circumstances, yawning and stretching may be considered part of the five classes of vibratory movements. When yawning occurs during attacks of fever and other diseases, it appears caused by sudden, strong contractions in the membranes of the mouth, throat, trachea and esophagus, whereas stretching appears caused by skin contractions.

Surprisingly, very few authors evoked yawning in animals or children. Charles Porée (1685–1770) spoke about yawning during a public session of the Académie des Belles-Lettres de Caen in 1756 where he observed [30]:

Birds yawn, just as man and several other animals do, but their yawning is different from ours. The lower part of the bird's beak is stable, whereas the upper part is mobile through a hinge connecting the bones of the bird's head to its beak. Our upper jaw is fixed, the lower jaw is mobile and moves with the temporal bones. When man yawns, the lower part of the mouth opens; while the mechanism differs, nature's intention is the same and reaches the same objective. The rest of this observation has mere curiosity value. We yawn when we are born; the first infant to be born set the example. This movement cannot be attributed to worry, as the infant knows the society he enters. Hunger and sleepiness are not the immediate cause; food will be administered through a new channel. So at first yawning has to be related to the change the infant experiences as he begins to breathe and thereafter, to the new course the blood works its way through. It can also be seen as a sign of weariness caused by the fatigue of birth and the new oscillation of the humors. All these changes are admirable and show a providence worthy of our deepest esteem. Nonetheless, one could complain that birth as well as death are difficult, and life is often less tiresome.

Joseph Raulin (1708–1784) tried to classify the nervous disorders of the ladies he treated at the court of Louis XV [31]. In his *Traité des affections vaporeuses du sexe* ('*Treatise on Vaporous Affections of the Female Sex*'), he compared spasms and convulsions and used the expression of the period – vapors – to describe what would later be known as hysteria, characterized by Paul Briquet (1796–1881) and Jean Baptiste Louyer-Villermay (1776–1838) at the beginning of the 19th century:

A woman experiences anxieties, yawning, hiccups, spasms and irregular movements in her nerves, of which she complains bitterly; her family, friends and neighbors respond with indifference. This is a case of vapors. These light vapors progress imperceptibly, the patient becomes sad, she sheds tears, or she seems cheerful, she uses expressions that are not understood, or she says pretty things, she laughs, she sings, or she alternates tears and laughter, always being beside herself. We laugh as she does, attributing this to the vapors.

History does not remember the name of Jean-Férapie Dufieu [32], yet he wrote a treatise of physiology for students, published in Lyon in 1763, in which he compiled the knowledge of his times in a literary style long forgotten in our modern manuals:

> When we wake, we yawn, stretch our arms, we are more agile, our spirit is more vivacious. Since the nervous juices do not flow through the muscles during sleep, all fibers are sluggish. Thus we have to contract them all, to open the passage for the nervous juices that have filtered into the brain, or to bring them into these parts. In addition, since the movement of blood through the muscles is sluggish, its course has to be hastened; this is done by contraction where the muscles enter when the limbs are stretched. Yawning has the same cause. These nervous juices that enter into the muscles, and that have gathered up in large quantities, make us more agile, because the soul can send a large amount into the nerves to move the body parts.

This colorful description is close to many of our current concepts at the start of the 21st century!

In 1767, Achille Le Vacher de la Feutrie compiled a dictionary of surgery [33], in which he returned to the concepts of Sanctorius and de Gorter:

> Imperceptibly we render a large quantity of perspirable matter when nature causes yawning and limb extension. We are more prone to yawning immediately after sleep than at other times, because a larger quantity of this perspirable matter escapes through the pores of the skin than at other times. The increase in contraction following this affluence causes the retention of perspirable matter in the passages of the skin; and that is the reason for the irritations that precede yawning and limb extension. During those movements all membranes of the body are shaken, their fibers are spread and the retained matter can escape.

Following Sydenham in England, François Boissier de Sauvages (1706–1767) [34], a famous practitioner at the University of Montpellier, tried to classify diseases using a methodology inspired by Linnaeus in the natural sciences, who generated great interest in taxonomy during that time. Boissier published a large body of work on different subject matters, but his *Nosologie Méthodique ou distribution des maladies en classes, en genres et en espèces* ('*Methodical Nosology* or *Assignment* of *Diseases* to *Classes*, *Types* and *Species*') remains his most famous work [35]:

> Through the full and deep breathing that accompanies yawning, all pulmonary vesicles dilate, blood circulation in the lungs accelerates, the viscera of the lower abdomen compress, the eyes water, saliva flows abundantly, the hearing muffles, a sort of buzzing is felt inside the head, the Eustachian tube dilates, talking is impossible, perspiration increases, the soul experiences a sort of exquisite pleasure, and the person becomes more energized and more alert.

Boissier goes on to review different kinds of pathological yawning: during hemorrhages as during fevers yawning announces a fatal outcome, whereas 'stomach yawning' bears witness to indigestion and disgust. He also describes vapors accompanied by yawning, which he qualifies as hysterical.

Samuel Tissot (1728–1797) returned to practice in Lausanne after having studied in Montpellier. As a physician to prominent figures between 1750 and 1797, he was consulted all over Europe, often by correspondence. His archives contained all the medical correspondence, including prescriptions, that he conducted with his patients. His *Avis au peuple sur sa santé* ('*Notice to the General Public Concerning Their Health*') was a true early-day bestseller [35–37], translated into 12 languages and published in 17 editions. It was the first medical book written for the general public in the vernacular language. However, above all, Tissot is the author of the first treatise on neurology, *Traité des nerfs et de leurs maladies* (*'Treatise on Nerves and Nervous Disorders'*, 1768–1770), the first volume of which is entitled *Traité de l'épilepsie* ('Treatise on epilepsy'). He attributed the transmission of information from one body part to another to a fluid circulating in the nerves that he called 'sympathies':

Such is the admirable constitution of man and animal, that those parts with seemingly different functions are however intertwined such that they all more or less influence one another [...] But aside from this general harmony, there are different parts that have a more direct connection, that are linked by different means, such that the state of one has a pronounced influence on the state of another, or is at least altered by the changes that it experiences; this is due to the Greek sympathia and the Latin consensus; and sometimes the effect is much more pronounced on the part in sympathy than on the part originally affected. [...] Since specific sympathies depend on nerves that have closer connections, weak causes can set them into motion; stronger causes are needed to bring about the well pronounced effects of general sympathy. All men are not equally subject to sympathies, because the nervous nature is not equally sensitive in all; hence, the same cause that brings about the most pronounced sympathies in one person, causes none in another; the corresponding action is limited to its centre, because the nerves of that person are less sensitive. It is strictly to the general consensus that we must attribute this imitative force that obliged Monro to repeat all that he saw being done. M. Whytt attributes yawning and involuntary vomiting to it; but I nonetheless do not know whether simple physical consensus is capable of generating these phenomena by itself.

Robert Whytt (1714–1766), a medical professor in Edinburgh, is known for having described tubercular meningitis. His explanation of 'sensations' (sensitivity) in involuntary movements makes him a forerunner in the area of reflexes, just as his interest in the effect of emotions during diseases makes him the father of psychosomatic pathology [38, 39]:

The different parts of our body receive from nerves not only the power to feel and move, but also a very specific sympathy that is either general and spreads out over the entire animal system, or particular, meaning that it is mainly exerted between certain parts. Whether we want to or not, we close both our eyelids every time there is a threat to one of our eyes. A sudden bright light striking our eyes sometimes causes blindness. Hippocrates observed that the sudden sight of a snake can make the face go pale. When a hungry person sees food he likes, he experiences a more abundant secretion of saliva than before having seen the object. Yawning and vomiting often occur by the simple sight or sound of someone yawning or vomiting. In this work on nervous disorders, I will mainly examine those that have the effect of a weak, delicate and unusual nervous constitution; and in this category I place the majority of symptoms that physicians have commonly described as windy, spastic, hypochondriacal, hysterical and vaporous [...] Those that can suddenly be felt in the entire body or that travel through it; shivers, a feeling of coldness in certain parts as if water were being poured on them; at other times, an unusual feeling of fire [...] Heart palpitations, rapidly changing pulse, most often natural, sometimes unusually slow, and other times quick or frequent, more often faint that strong, and in certain cases irregular or intermittent [...] A dry cough with breathing troubles, or a convulsion or tightening of the bronchi, an accident that may come back periodically, yawning, hiccups, frequent sighing, a feeling of suffocation or constriction that seems to be caused by a lump or large object lodged in the throat, fits of crying and convulsive laughter.

Erasmus Darwin (1731–1802) is famous for being the grandfather of Charles and the author of *Zoonomia or The Laws of Organic Life* (1794) [40]. In this work, he is the first to describe the movement of a paralyzed arm in a hemiplegic during yawning:

These involuntary motions are often seen in paralytic limbs, which are at the same time completely disobedient to the will.

L'art de connaître les hommes par la physionomie (*'The Art of Understanding Men by Their Physiognomy'*, 1775–1778) by Gaspard Lavater (1741–1800) was the result of a philosophical movement dating back to Antiquity that consisted of deciphering an individual's personality from his facial features [41]. Lavater's chapter on yawning was particularly novel:

During the most passionate moments, the jaw often has an involuntary movement just as during moments when the soul is unaffected; pain, pleasure and boredom also cause yawning, but it is true that vivid yawning is a convulsion that is very prompt during pain or pleasure, whereas the yawning of boredom shows its character by the slow pace at which it occurs.

19th Century: Yawning and Hysteria

François Magendie (1783–1855) demonstrated the discoveries of Charles Bell, who distinguished the ventral roots as being motor nerves and the dorsal roots as being sensory nerves. Magendie defended his thesis on 27 March 1808: *Essai sur l'usage du voile du palais* (*'Essay on the Use of the Soft Palate'*) which included a novel chapter on yawning [42]:

Yawning, classified by physiologists among inhalation phenomena, has not been sufficiently studied in my opinion. It is generally considered a long inhalation made necessary by the slowing of the circulation upon waking, before sleep and in melancholy passions such as boredom, etc. But if we attentively examine yawning, we recognize that it is often composed of several inhalations and exhalations. At other times it occurs after inhalation, thus during exhalation. In certain rare cases we yawn without breathing in or out; this strongly suggests that yawning mainly consists in the pandiculation of the masseter, temporal and pterygoid muscles and in the prolonged contraction of the submandibular muscles. I do not completely exclude the purpose given by physiologists to yawning, but I think it must be seen as accessory. Another reason makes me persist in this idea: yawning is almost always accompanied by the pandiculation of other muscles in the body, and important muscles such as the masseter and pterygoid muscles must necessarily take part in the well-being resulting from this elongation. Do we not observe in the jaw muscles the two kinds of pandiculation seen in the trunk and the limbs? In one, the most frequent kind, we extend the limbs, we arch the trunk backwards, the flexors are elongated, the extensors contracted. In the other, the opposite happens, meaning that the trunk and the limbs are in the greatest degree of flexion possible: the extensors are elongated, the flexors are strongly contracted. We find these two kinds of pandiculation in the muscles of the lower jaw during simple yawning: the levators are elongated, the depressors contracted; in a particular state that has not yet been described, the levator muscles as well as all facial muscles enter into a violent contraction and we experience a sensation that is perfectly identical to the one felt during yawning.

Julien César Legallois (1770–1814) was a pioneer in experimental physiology. In 1813 he published his *Expériences sur les principes de la vie* (*'Experiments on the Principles of Life'*) in which he described sectioning the spinal cord of live rabbits in several locations, which allowed him to place the respiratory centers in the brainstem [43]. He reported the occurrence of yawning numerous times and considered it as a ventilatory movement:

Whatever the origin of respiratory nerves, the motive force for the respiratory function is undoubtedly in the brain. Were new proof needed, the yawning I observed after sectioning the spinal cord provides us with evidence that appears irrefutable.

Yawning clearly depends on the same motive force as spontaneous inhalation; yawning is the remains, and to some extent the vestiges of this inhalation.

Auguste Landre-Beauvais (1772–1840) created a new genre by proposing one of the first books on medical semiology: *Traité des signes des maladies* (*'Treatise on the Signs of Diseases'*, 1815). He described yawning associated with diverse pathological states [44]:

Yawning generally occurs before febrile shivering. It sometimes occurs in ataxic fevers and frequently precedes eruptions and hemorrhages. Attacks of gout, hysteria or hypochondria are often presaged by continuous yawning. Frequent yawning is sometimes observed during early pregnancy. Yawning is a phenomenon that occurs after serious injuries, excessive evacuation and internal inflammations; when accompanied by serious symptoms, it is a very worrisome sign. Frequent yawning during ataxic fevers may be considered very dangerous, particularly in connection with other phenomena that precede weakness. The same is true for yellow fever, the plague, and phlegmasia complicated by ataxic fever. Frequent yawning sometimes occurs in women during childbirth, indicating that the delivery will be difficult and that the mother's strength is oppressed or weakened. A feeling of weariness and heaviness in the limbs and less lively sensations immediately precede yawning. It is followed by increased cheerfulness and vivacity. The pulse becomes quicker and the temperature often increases. The secretion of tears and saliva is more abundant. If we relate these phenomena to what preceded the yawning – fatigue, boredom, an exterior cold – it seems that the objective of this effort is to improve the circulation in the lungs where the air flow has encountered obstacles produced by either spasm or plethora.

The first medical encyclopedic dictionary of the 19th century was managed by Charles-Louis-Fleury Panckoucke (1780–1844) and published in 60 volumes from 1812 to 1822. He solicited the great medical minds of his time such as Alibert, Pinel, Esquirol, Laënnec, Desgenettes and Larrey. This dictionary, including more than 4,000 bibliographic records and just over 200 illustrations, was an attempt to summarize the medical knowledge of the time, at the dawn of clinical medicine and anatomical pathology. The dictionary was a large commercial success, a source of wealth for its sponsor and a far-reaching vehicle for French medical thinking [45]. The entry on yawning was novel because it evoked yawning in animals and described fetal yawning, never before reported:

The Latin term for yawning comes from oscitatio; in French, bâillement is derived from the Latin balare, to bleat. Yawning consists of a large inhalation occurring slowly, and in general with wide opening of the jaws, followed by a prolonged exhalation, often accompanied by a muted noise. It is generally thought to be caused by a problem with pulmonary circulation. This opinion, while not being backed by any positive fact, does appear likely: almost all causes of yawning coincide with a certain weakness of the entire system, which could very well produce the problem we are discussing; the causes are boredom, sleepiness, fatigue, hunger, and the malaise preceding intermittent fevers, etc. Animals put into the pneumatic machine, those that are placed in non-breathable air, yawn several times before dying. A fetus taken alive from its mother's womb by caesarean operation yawns as well. Finally, it seems that damage to the pulmonary tissue can cause frequent yawning. In many cases this phenomenon seems related to the state of the stomach rather than to state of the lungs, which are only affected sympathetically; in this way, difficult digestion or a simple stomach pain, whatever the cause, is accompanied by repeated yawning. This incident can also be purely spasmodic, as observed in women affected by hysteria, or in individuals with convulsive diseases. Yawning is, to a certain extent, an involuntary act. We can overcome the action of muscles tightening to lower the jaw by contracting their antagonists; we can moderate the exhalation that ends yawning and prevent its accompanying noise. But the long inhalation that constitutes yawning itself cannot be suppressed, undoubtedly because the agent of this inhalation, the diaphragm, receives part of its nerves from the system of ganglia, as M. Roux has noted. Bichat suspected that the object of this involuntary act is to renew the air contained in the lungs more completely than can be achieved by ordinary inhalation, and thus give way to greater absorption of oxygen.

François-Joseph Double (1776–1842), famous during his time and a founding member of the Académie de Médecine, also published a treatise on semiology and disease in 1817: *Séméiologie générale ou traité des signes et de leur valeur dans les maladies* [46]. In his work, he summarized the same findings as Landre-Beauvais:

> A rapid consideration of the mechanism of yawning clearly suggests its degree of influence on the system. Its importance cannot be denied if we think about the general state that precedes and follows it, for example, the kind of stupor and torpor that prepares the way and the weariness and weakness we feel beforehand, in contrast to the pleasant sensation that follows and the relaxation and well-being it procures. By reflecting on these diverse subjects, we find the indication for most of the signs that experience has attached to yawning. […] Pandiculation consists of successive stretching of all muscles accompanied by a pleasant sensation and generally followed by yawning. […] Pandiculation is a very positive sign leading into convalescence, but if it continues and persists relentlessly, it indicates a deterioration. During the course of a disease, pandiculation is always salutary; it signals the favorable state of the vital forces and the resistance with which nature fights the effect of the disease.

During the same period, at the age of 22 years, Anthelme Richerand (1779–1840), known for his quarrels with Dupuytren, published *Nouveaux éléments de physiologie* (*'New Elements of Physiology'*) [47]. This important compilation of writings from the period lacked originality but possessed a style that made it a highly successful teaching tool, as this account confirms:

> This work brought charm and beauty to our school years. It was a delightful introduction to the austere study of medicine; the reading could be considered light, but it seemed to sprinkle the subject's first paths with flowers.

The article on yawning demonstrates this:

> We also yawn upon waking, in order to lift the thorax muscles to an appropriate degree for respiration, which is always slower, less frequent and deeper during sleep than during the waking state. Due to a similar need, waking in all animals is marked by pandiculation, a muscular action in which the muscles seem to accommodate the contractions that the movements dictate. The crowing of the cock and the agitation of its wings serve the same purpose. Finally, the same necessity leads the numerous flocks of birds that inhabit our woods to warble endlessly at sunrise and fill the air with harmonious song, in which the poet hears the joyous hymn by which the feathered populace celebrates the return of the god of light!

Nicolas Adelon (1782–1862) was the author of a long article devoted to yawning in the *Dictionnaire de Médecine* published from 1829 to 1836 [48]. He expanded on the respiratory theory of yawning, helping to ensure its 150 years of success:

> In the state of health, yawning occurs in a vacuum, in a situation where there is no renewal of fresh air, because in these cases there is not enough air, or the air contains less oxygen, and we try to compensate by introducing a large amount of air to where it is lacking. This is why yawning is a precursory phenomenon of all gradual asphyxiations. We yawn when sleep approaches, because the momentary paralysis that seizes all muscles in the body also seems to seize the respiratory

muscles, which results in a temporary decrease in the frequency of inhalation. Since the circulation has continued in the meantime, and as a result has carried the same quantity of venous blood to the lungs to be transformed into arterial blood, there is not enough air to perform this conversion, and a small amount of venous blood remains in the lungs, slightly blocking pulmonary circulation: yawning thus occurs automatically to introduce a larger quantity of air, the quantity needed to arterialize the leftover venous blood and restore balance. Yawning occurs in all circumstances where we see this accumulation of venous blood in the lungs, this blockage of pulmonary circulation. It is thus considered a physiological remedy for dissipating this engorgement, and its full accomplishment is followed by a sensation of well-being. Judging from this feeling, the outside air introduced into the lungs by yawning could be considered to overcome the obstacle blocking the circulation in these organs. We also yawn during the first moments of waking, because inhalation occurs in a different mode than during sleep, and in the passage from one mode to the other, there is a momentary decrease in inhalation, due to an imbalance in the amount of air introduced and the quantity of venous blood to be transformed into arterial blood. The result is a slight pulmonary engorgement, leading to the phenomenon necessary clear it.

During the same period, John M. Good (1764–1827) explained yawning and pandiculation in *The Study of Medicine with a Physiological System of Nosology* in England [49]. Taking a very different approach from his contemporaries on the continent, he never evoked the ventilatory mechanism, but saw yawning as simple muscular work necessary for the balance between extensors and flexors. These notions come close to modern-day physiological observations.

In 1861, Adolphe Dureau de la Malle (1777–1851) published a dissertation on the development of intellectual faculties in wild and domesticated animals in the *Annales de Sciences Naturelles* [50]. He reported having such close ties to his dog that the latter started yawning when he saw his master yawn! Present day authors Joly-Mascheroni and Senju published a study in 2008 that comes to similar conclusions [51].

François Broussais (1772–1838) broke away entirely from his contemporaries and predecessors in his *Traité de physiologie appliqué à la pathologie* (*'Treatise on Physiology Applied to Pathology'*), published in 1834 [52]:

If we wish to study the mechanism of yawning, which can be considered as the first sign and main phenomenon of boredom, either moral or physical, we will encounter serious problems. Yawning has been related to the need to breathe, or considered a means to renew the air stagnating in the lungs after respiration has slowed for some time. This is an error – one must only be a practitioner to know with certainty that dyspnea alone never produces yawning. [...] The lungs seem to be much less influenced by yawning than the stomach ... [If] the need for air is not the principal cause of this deep aspiration, then what can its purpose be? Could it be to swallow air, and to cure an ill stomach?

This novel approach did not generate much response and the ventilatory theory persisted.

John Abercrombie (1780–1844), a Scottish physician, published *Pathological and Practical Researches on the Diseases of the Brain and Spinal Cord* in 1828 [53], which was translated into French in 1832. He described the strange phenomenon encountered in certain hemiplegics where the paralyzed arm moves up towards the mouth simultaneous to yawning. This occurrence disappeared as soon as the paralysis subsided.

In 1842, Pierre-Marie Flourens (1794–1867) gave a clear explanation of motor automatisms and their coordination – Recherches expérimentales sur les propriétés et les fonctions du système nerveux dans les animaux vertébrés (*'Experimental Research on Nervous System Functioning in Vertebrates'*) [54]:

The spinal cord is restricted to linking muscular contractions, the first elements of all movement, into complex movements. Although the spinal cord is the point of departure for almost all nerves determining these contractions and movements, it is not the seat of the admirable power to coordinate them into specific movements: jumping, flying, walking, running, resting, etc.; or inhaling, shouting, yawning, etc. This power resides in the cerebellum for the first group, in the spinal bulb for the second group. There is one last consideration to note. The movements of respiration, shouting, yawning, etc., are commonly called involuntary, whereas locomotive movements are called voluntary.

Louis Delasiauve (1804–1893) and Théodore Herpin (1799–1865) are associated with the detailed description of the different types of epilepsy, which include generalized and partial seizures. They described prodromes warning the patient of an imminent seizure, notably repeated yawning. These symptoms are currently attributed to partial temporal seizures [55–57].

End of the 19th Century: Is Yawning a Reflex?

Jean-Louis Brachet (1789–1858), an eminent physiologist in Lyon, was the first to contest the respiratory role of yawning [58]:

Yawning is generally defined as a large, deep inhalation occurring slowly that moves the lower jaw, the hyoid bone and the larynx considerably downward. It is followed by a prolonged exhalation accompanied by a particular muted noise. Yawning is attributed to the need to renew air in the lungs, or to introduce a larger quantity of air to supply the blood with more oxygen, because the flow is blocked and oxygen is consequently lacking. Or yawning is attributed to a feeling of malaise arising in the back of the throat, in the upper part of the neck. We do not share this view. We do not consider the phenomenon to be limited to this convulsive contraction of the facial and neck muscles, nor to this larger volume of air that it sends through the airways. Yawning is not a purely local phenomenon pertaining exclusively to respiration: it is a general phenomenon pertaining to the complete system. [...] We therefore think yawning, as well as pandiculation, occurs when the brain, alerted by the torpor seizing the system, tries to prevent the consequences by soliciting acts of excitation and arousal; thus all muscles contract, the locomotive as well as the respiratory muscles. This general contraction is already a means of stimulation.

Almire Lepelletier de la Sarthe (1790–1880), a proponent of physiognomy which Johann-Casper Lavater developed in 1775, largely surpassed his master with his reprehensible words [59–61]:

When yawning is customary, we can assume the following about the subject: limited intelligence, without initiative, slow and lazy mind, inactive, soft character, weak, indolent, timid, indifferent, melancholic, boring, incapable of vigorous resolution or undertaking a long, difficult or perilous enterprise, at times clever and cunning, and given to contemplating theft and fraud in his dealings.

In 1865, Jules-Bernard Luys (1828–1897) published *Recherches sur le système nerveux cérébro-spinal, sa structure, ses fonctions et ses maladies* (Studies on the Cerebrospinal Nervous System, Its Structure, Functions and Diseases' [62]). He described the central grey nuclei, giving his name to one of them, and postulated on their physiological role, which had never been studied before his time. He developed novel ideas concerning yawning as well:

> Although not extensively discussed, it is a common observation that when the brain cells start to become inactive, the medullary regions of the spinal axis with immediate control over the respiratory apparatus are altered in their functioning. Everyone knows that yawning is a premonitory sign that the conditions of diurnal functional activity in the nervous system have ceased to be what they previously were. What is yawning if not an involuntary inhalation indicating that the innervation of automatic activity acquires a predominate influence in the medullary region, following retrocession of the cerebral influx, and that at this precise point of the spinal axis, a sort of interregnum occurs and a disturbance of the original stimulus. In addition, the highly characteristic rhythm of the respiratory movements during the period of brain collapse, their well-measured succession and their overtly automatic nature lead us to believe that they are no longer controlled by the same centres of innervation that supply them during the waking state.

We have now reached the end of the 19th century, which was dominated by the work of Jean-Martin Charcot (1825–1893) and his students Charles Féré (1852–1907) and Georges Gilles de la Tourette (1857–1904). The most famous observation of pathological yawning was presented by J.M. Charcot on Tuesday, 23 October 1888 [63]. His young 17-year-old patient yawned 8 times per minute, or 480 times per hour, only interrupted by sleep; she had generalized epileptic seizures, complete anosmia and binasal hemianopsia. Reporting this observation in the *La Nouvelle Iconographie de la Salpêtrière* in 1890, Gilles de la Tourette specified that she had been amenorrheic for nearly a year, but he did not indicate whether she was examined for galactorrhea. And yet J.M. Charcot noted: 'After what I have told you, you have undoubtedly surmised that we are in the domain of hysteria.' If we may criticize the master 120 years later, J.M. Charcot's young patient was most likely suffering from a prolactinoma compressing her optic chiasma and her hypothalamus. Surprisingly, J.M. Charcot continues his discussion without evoking any criticism:

> Physiologically we affirm that this is an automatic act, required by a certain degree of anoxemia, a need for oxygenation of the nervous centers.

In the third volume of *La Nouvelle Iconographie de la Salpêtrière* (1890), Gilles de la Tourette added four other observations involving abnormal movements and convulsions attributed to hysteria [64]. It is difficult to establish an exact diagnosis, but an organic pathology involving the thalamus or hypothalamus seems probable, such as a tumor with intracranial hypertension or a chronic tic disorder. In 1895, Gilles de la Tourette reviewed and commented on these cases again in his *Traité de l'hystérie en trois volumes* (*'Treatise of Hysteria in Three Volumes'*), justifying what he believed to be their hysterical origin [65]. Lastly, in 1905, Féré published a report on yawning to the Société de Biologie that describes his efforts to measure muscular force, observing its decrease after yawning [66].

Paolo Mantegazza [67] (1831–1910) was an Italian psychologist and author of *La physionomie et l'expression des sentiments* (*'Facial Characteristics and the Expression of Sentiment'*). He was the first to report:

> Yawning expresses a wide variety of things, such as hunger, thirst and, especially in women, the need for physical love; but in the expression of pain it is a characteristic element of boredom.

In 1891, Henrietta Russell, an American from New York, published a book called *Yawning* [68]. In this, she described natural gymnastics, comparable to contemporary relaxation, and explained the benefits of yawning, which results from relaxation and produces a feeling of release and well-being. She has since gained a following, and a thesis was dedicated to this topic in 2006 in France.

20th Century

The year 1901 is key in the study of yawning. René Trautmann (1875–1956) defended his doctoral thesis – *Le bâillement* – in Bordeaux under the direction of Paul Vergely [69]. It is the first of three dissertations on this topic presented in France during the 20th century, and by far the most interesting. Trautmann, educated in a military medical school, spent his entire military career as a physician in Africa. He produced ethnological studies that were marked by the colonizing spirit of the period, in addition to a few short stories based on his travels. His thesis presents a very rich historical perspective and one that is still very useful. Trautmann described the activation of the facial muscles and respiratory channels in detail, as none of his predecessors had, and concluded that yawning improves blood oxygenation. He reviewed the different theories explaining the contagiousness of yawning and proposed that:

> Yawning falls into the category of occurrences reinforced by habit and favored by moral depression. When the mind concentrates, when we are very attentively listening to a story, we do not yawn, even if one or more people engage in this act. Yawning is a purely imitative phenomenon, as are the gestures and involuntary facial movements executed by many individuals attending a speech or declamation. Depending on the subject, more frequent yawning is the result of a greater tendency towards instinctive imitation.

Trautmann accepted the idea that yawning is involuntary but challenged the historical writings he cited by proposing a method to trigger yawning at will:

> [For] some time we have observed that we can willfully effectuate complete yawning by means of a particular mechanism; several of our colleagues, who are medical students, have reached the same conclusion. One need only tighten the subhyoid muscles vigorously while inhaling slowly and profoundly. The lower jaw is dropped down and pushed forward, and there is a buzzing in the ears: yawning takes place.

Trautmann thoroughly reviewed all forms of pathological yawning and added personal observations of a rapid succession of yawns during shivering at the onset of fever. A long chapter describes yawning in pregnant women, especially during puerperal fever or delivery accompanied by hemorrhaging. It is completed by Trautmann's own observations. In his conclusion, he writes:

> While yawning always occurs in the same manner, it can be considered – as a muscular act and depending on the case in which it occurs – as a particular type of reflex: (a) an exclusively spinal reflex, (b) a mesencephalic reflex or (c) a cerebral and cortical reflex.

At the end of his thesis, Trautmann challenges the ventilatory theory, which does not explain all the clinical cases he presents, and his work suggests the existence of neurological mechanisms that trigger yawning. Trautmann thus appears to be the first modern-day thinker on yawning.

In 1905, André Vigouroux and Paul Juquelier wrote a book entitled *La contagion mentale* (*'Mental Contagion'*) [70]. They saw yawning as a reflex, which made it contagious by nature. In particular, they developed a hypothesis that became successful under the term 'théorie de l'esprit' (mind theory). It stated that by involuntarily mimicking the gestures, actions and emotions of others, we acquire the ability to decode the feelings of the person we observe. Interest in this theory was renewed with the discovery of mirror neurons at the end of the 20th century [71]:

> [The] sight of coordinated, rhythmic actions that have become reflexes for those who perform them, provokes in onlookers motor reactions that are perfectly involuntary but also rhythmic and that represent a rough reproduction of the perceived acts.

In 1916, F.H. Pike from Columbia University in New York proposed a comprehensive review in the *Journal of Heredity*. Taking account of animals and human fetuses, Pike rethought the origin of yawning, discussing both the influence of hunger and the need to fight an enemy [72].

In *The Lancet* (21 January 1905), John Hughlings Jackson described a personal observation. While performing a funduscopy on a patient, he suddenly observed a retinal paleness attributed to an arteriolar spasm that was quickly followed by yawning, which restored the appearance of the retina [73].

The period following World War I was marked by a significant epidemic of encephalitis lethargica, also called von Economo disease [74]. In addition to the lethargic forms that were often fatal, or the curable forms that left the patient with Parkinson's disease and abnormal movements (oculogyric crises), a rarer form of encephalitis manifested itself through stubborn and fatal insomnia, very often accompanied by a rapid succession of yawns. In 1921, Jean Sicard and André Paraff published a case associated with uncontrollable laughter, comparable to gelastic epilepsy [75]. In 1922, Gabrielle Lévy, a student of Pierre Marie and Jean Lhermitte dedicated her thesis to this topic in France [76]. At the same time, Arthur Hall in England [77], Smith E. Jelliffe in the USA [78], Raymond de Saussure in Switzerland [79], and Georges Guillain and Pierre Mollaret in Paris [80] all collected observations in which yawning can be interpreted as abnormal movement, similar to tics and relaxation behavior at the end of involuntary episodes of hyperventilation.

Edouard Claparède (1873–1940) was a Genevan physician and psychologist. One of his specialties was child psychology. In a journal for teachers entitled *L'Educateur*, he published an article in 1924 [81] that drew on the work of the German Valentin Dumpert in 1921 [82]. He noted that yawning results from a massive contraction of the diaphragm and is part of pandiculation, rather than being directly tied to breathing. He was the first to overturn the paradigm of ventilatory yawning, pioneering today's neuromuscular theory in which yawning has a diencephalic origin:

Yawning is only incomprehensible when considered alone. On the contrary, it becomes clearer if we see it as part of a more general reflex, the reflex of stretching. It is well known that yawning hardly ever occurs without general stretching of the body. This is striking in certain animals, such as dogs or cats. It is also evident in small infants, and very often in adults.

Through self-observation, Dumpert noted that voluntary stretching activates yawning (this is easy to reproduce). He also observed that yawning evokes associated movements in hemiplegics; they present extension in their paralyzed limbs that lasts throughout the yawn. Claparède was convinced that these associated movements were part of the stretching reflex: 'When one of our listeners yawns, can we assume he is tired of listening to us, when on the contrary, he may be doing his best to keep listening?'. Yawning thus became a means of stimulating vigilance, a true revolution!

In 1937 Paul Delmas-Marsallet presented an article entitled 'Le signe du bâillement dans les lésions du cerveau frontal' ('Yawning in frontal brain damage') in the journal *Oto-Neuro-Ophtalmologie* [83]. He described five observations of uncontrollable yawning resulting from either frontal hematomas or frontal tumors. He proposed that uncontrollable yawning was a clinical sign of intercranial hypertension, which remains true.

In 1946, Paul Heusner published the first summary article in English in *Physiological Review*. Phylogenesis emerged for the first time [84]. Heusner precisely described different durations and scientifically measured daily timescales. He proposed that the brainstem and basal ganglia were responsible for yawning, based on yawning in anencephalic newborns and in hemiplegics during brachial parakinesis.

In 1958, Jean Barbizet published a large compilation of data and historical information in French and English [85], together with the first radioscopic measurements, which he had taken, of pharyngolaryngeal expansion during yawning. He thus showed that during the culmination of yawning, pharyngolaryngeal diameter is multiplied by four. He also described the first works of P. Passouant, who triggered experimental yawning in cats by electrostimulation of the hypothalamus. In addition to mentioning involuntary parakinesis in the paralyzed arm of a hemiplegic, he reported the unusual observation of D. Furtado, in which passive movement in the paralyzed arm of a polio patient triggered yawning, which has never been reported since [86].

In 1962, A. Montagu wrote an article in the *JAMA* that has since been frequently quoted. He proposed that yawning stimulated vigilance, while attributing lowered vigilance to insufficient brain oxygenation [87].

J. Boudouresque attempted to summarize knowledge on yawning for the *Encyclopédie Médico-Chirurgicale* in 1965 [88]. Returning to the old concept of yawning as a modified respiratory act, he clearly identified it as originating in the diencephalon and the brainstem. After cataloguing all the causes of excessive yawning, he concluded: 'Yawning is the most suggestive sign of mesodiencephalic distress. It has considerable prognostic value as a synonym of gravity.'

The age of pharmacology began in 1963 with publications on the experimental activation of yawning, always associated with erection and often with stretching of the limbs in rats, cats and mangabey monkeys. In the *Annals of the New York Academic of Sciences*, Ferrari et al. [89] published the results of intracerebral injection of ACTH, a pituitary hormone stimulating the secretion of cortisol and other adrenocorticoids. ACTH, a peptide with 41 amino acids, is produced from a precursor (proopiomelanocortin) and acts on the paraventricular nucleus of the hypothalamus; however, proopiomelanocortin is also the precursor of other hormones, such as α-MSH (which stimulates melanogenesis). These hormones were shown to activate yawning after cortical injection [89].

The central role of the paraventricular nucleus in the hypothalamus was identified in 1980 by the work of W. Ferrari, A. Argiolas, and M.R. Melis in Italy, as well as R. Urba-Holmgren and B. Holmgren in Mexico [90]. This transformed the approach to the dopaminergic and cholinergic systems in the brain.

During the 1980s and 1990s, American psychologists R. Provine and R. Baenninger published the first scientific work on the behavioral study of yawning, based on observations of their students [91, 92]. Ethnologists B.L. Deputte in France [93] and F. Troisi in the Netherlands [94], working with no apparent connection or consultation, described different types of yawning in non-human primates, notably testosterone-dependent yawning in dominant males.

Today, at the start of the 21st century, the neurohormonal mechanisms appear to be established, making yawning a marker of activity in D_3 dopamine receptors. The study of 'contagious' yawning offers an example of non-verbal language that is part of the theory of mind. Observations such as the lack of yawning in autistic children together with brain imaging studies are changing the neuropsychological approach to involuntary decoding of emotions, bringing yawning closer to empathy.

Having been associated with forced ventilation for centuries, yawning has become an emotional stereotypy exteriorizing homeostatic phenomena in the systems controlling arousal, hunger and sexuality.

References

1 Mencken HL: Treatise on Right and Wrong. New York, Knopf, 1934.

2 Coxe JR: The Writings of Hippocrates and Galen Epitomized from the Original Latin Translations. Vol: Of Flatus. Philadelphia, Lindsay and Blakiston, 1846.

3 Coxe JR: The Writings of Hippocrates and Galen Epitomized from the Original Latin Translations. Vol: On the Nature of the Bones: On the Reduction of Fractures and Luxations. Philadelphia, Lindsay and Blakiston, 1846.

4 Littré E: Œuvres d'Hippocrate. Paris, Baillière, 1853.

5 Hippocrate: Des vents, De Flatibus. Oeuvres complètes (texte établi par J. Jouanna). Paris, Les belles Lettres, 2003, vol 5.

6 Pline l'Ancien: Naturalis Historiae Libri XXXVII. Ex editione Gabrielis Brotier. Volumen Tertium. Londini, Imprimente Valpy, 1826.

7 Lapehn JD: De oscitatione in enixu. Thèse soutenue devant JG. Roederer. Göttingen, Litteris Pockwitzii et Barmeieri, 1758.

8 Sénèque: Une introduction, suivie de la lettre 70 des Lettres à Lucilius P. Veyne. Paris, Tallandier, 2007.

9 Oribase: Œuvres d'. Bussemaker et Daremberg. Paris, Imprimerie Impériale, 1858, vol 3.

10 Fernelii J: Universa medicina, cum notis, observationibus et remedÿs secretis. Van Heurne, Otto (dit Heurnius). Trajecti ad Rhenum, typis G. a Zijll et T. ab Ackersdijck, 1656.

11 Lommius ou Van Lom J: Medicinalium Observationim Librites. Antwerpioe, Sylvius, 1560.

12 Duffin J: Jodocus Lommius's Little Golden Book and the history of diagnostic semeiology. J Hist Med Allied Sci 2006;61:249–287.
13 Hoechstetter P: Rararum Observationum Medicinalium Decades tres continentes, historias medicas, theorica and practica varia. Augusta Vindelicorum, Aperger, 1624.
14 Dupleix S: La curiosité naturelle rédigée en questions. Paris, Sonnius, 1626.
15 Sanctorius S: La médecine statique ou l'art de conserver la santé par la transpiration, traduite en français par Le Breton. Paris, Briasson, 1726.
16 Eknoyan G: Santorio Sanctorius (1561–1636) – founding father of metabolic balance studies. Am J Nephrol 1999;19:226–233.
17 Descartes R: L'Homme et la formation du fœtus. Paris, Angot Ch, 1664.
18 Senerti D: Operum: Tomus Primus. Huguetan A, Sc. Lugduni, 1666.
19 Van Helmont JB: Les œuvres traitant de médecine et de physique, dans la traduction de J Le Conte. Lyon, Huguetan and Barbier, 1671.
20 Boerhaave H: Praelectiones Academicae. Göttingen, Vandenhoeck, 1739.
21 Beutler JB: De Oscitatione. Lipsiae, Fleischerl lib., 1685.
22 Hermann G: De Oscitatione et pandiculatione. Kohlesii Imp., 1720.
23 Brisseau P: Traité des mouvements simpathiques. Valenciennes, Henry Imp., 1692.
24 Cheyne G: The English Malady: Treatise of Nervous Diseases of all Kinds. London, Strahan Imp, 1733.
25 Gorter de J: De perspiratione insensibili, ed 2. Italica, Manfrè Imp. Patavii, 1755.
26 Haller von A: Elementa physiologiae corporis humani, ed 3. Lausanne, Pott Imp., 1777–1778.
27 Hartley D: Explication physique des sens, des idées et des mouvements tant volontaires qu'involontaires. Reims, Delaistre-Godet Lib., 1755.
28 Smith CU: David Hartley's newtonian neuropsychology. J Hist Behav Sci 1987;23:123–136.
29 Webb ME: The early medical studies and practice of Dr. David Hartley. Bull Hist Med 1989;63:618–636.
30 Porée CG: Essay sur le bâillement. Mémoire de l'Académie des Belles-Lettres de Caen, séance du 5 février 1756. Caen, 1757.
31 Raulin J: Traité des affections vaporeuses du sexe. Paris, Herissant Lib., 1758.
32 Dufieu JF: Traité de physiologie. Lyon, Jacquenod Fils. Lib., 1763.
33 Le Vacher de la Feutrie AF: Dictionnaire de chirurgie. Paris, Lacombe Lib., 1767.
34 Boissier de Sauvages de Lacroix F: Nosologica methodica sistens morborum classes. Amstelodami, Fratrum de Tournes, 1768.
35 Tissot S: Traité des nerfs et de leurs maladies. Paris, Didot Imp., 1778.
36 Tissot S: De la santé des gens de lettres. Paris, Didot Imp., 1769.
37 Karbowski K: Samuel Auguste Tissot (1728–1797). J Neurol 2001;248:1109–1110.
38 Whytt R: Traité des maladies nerveuses, hypochondriaques et hystériques. Paris, Didot Lib., 1777.
39 Pearce JM: Robert Whytt and the stretch reflex. J Neurol Neurosurg Psychiatry 1997;62:484.
40 Darwin E: Zoonomia or the Laws of Organic Life. London, J. Johnson, 1801.
41 Lavater CJ: L'art de connaitre les hommes par la physionomie. Paris, Depelafol Lib., 1820.
42 Magendie F: Essai sur le voile du palais, avec quelques propositions sur la fracture du cartilage des côtes. Thèse n° 21, soutenue le 27 mars 1808. Paris, Didot Jeune Imp., 1808.
43 Legallois JJC: Expériences sur le principe de la vie notamment sur celui des mouvemens du cœur, et sur le siège de ce principe. Paris, Chez d'Hautel, 1812.
44 Landre-Beauvais AJ: Sémiotique ou traité des signes des maladies. Paris, Brosson Lib., 1815.
45 Panckoucke CL: Dictionnaire des sciences médicales. Paris, Panckoucke, 1812.
46 Double FJ: Sémiologie générale ou traité des signes et de leur valeur dans les maladies. Paris, Croullebois Lib., 1817.
47 Richerand A: Elémens de physiologie. Paris, Caille et Ravier, 1817.
48 Adelon N: Dictionnaire de médecine et de chirurgie pratiques. Paris, Gabon, Méquignon-Marvis, Baillière, Crochard, 1829–1836.
49 Good JM: The Study of Medicine. London, Thomas and George Underwood, 1829.
50 Dureau de la Malle A: Annales des Sciences Naturelles. Paris, Crocahrd, 1831.
51 Joly-Mascheroni RM, Senju A, Shepherd AJ: Dogs catch human yawns. Biol Lett 2008;4:446–448.
52 Broussais F: Traité de physiologie appliquée à la pathologie. Paris, Baillière Lib., 1834.
53 Abercrombie J: Pathological and Practical Researches on Diseases of the Brain and the Spinal Cord. Edinburgh, Waugh and Innes, 1828.
54 Flourens PM: Recherches expérimentales sur les propriétés et fonctions du système nerveux dans les animaux vertébrés. Paris, Baillière, 1842.
55 Delasiauve L: Traité de l'épilepsie. Paris, Masson, 1854.
56 Herpin T: Des accès incomplets d'épilepsie. Paris, Baillière, 1867.
57 Eadie MJ: The epileptology of Théodore Herpin (1799–1865). Epilepsia 2002;43:1256–1261.
58 Brachet JL: Physiologie élémentaire de l'Homme. Paris et Savy Lib. Lyon, Germer-Baillière, 1855.

59 Lepelletier de la Sarthe A: Traité complet de physiognomonie. Paris, Masson, 1864.
60 Lavater CJ: L'art de connaitre les hommes par la physionomie. Paris, Depelafol Lib., 1820.
61 Dumont M: The social success of a false science: the physiognomy of Johann Kaspar Lavater. Actes Rech Sci Soc 1984;54:3–30.
62 Luys J: Recherches sur le système nerveux cérébrospinal, sa structure, ses fonctions et ses maladies. Paris, Baillière, 1865.
63 Charcot JM: Leçons du lardi à La Salpêtrière. Paris, Bureaux du Progrès Médical et Delahaye, 1887.
64 Gilles de la Tourette G, Huet, Guinon: Nouvelle Iconographie de La Salpêtrière. Paris, Lecrosnier et Babé, 1890, vol 3.
65 Gilles de la Tourette G: Traité clinique et thérapeutique de l'hystérie d'après l'enseignement de La Salpêtrière. Paris, Nourrit. Imp., 1895.
66 Féré C: Note sur le bâillement. C R Soc Biol (Paris) 1905;2:11–12.
67 Mantegazza P: La physionomie et l'expression des sentiments. Paris, Alcan, 1897.
68 Hovey R: Yawning (Delsarte Series No. 1). New York, US Book Company, 1891.
69 Trautmann A: Le bâillement. Thèse No. 40 soutenue le 20 décembre 1901. Bordeaux, Imp du Midi, 1901.
70 Vigouroux A et Juquelier P: La contagion mentale. Paris, Douin, 1905.
71 Rizzolatti G, Fogassi L, Gallese V: Neurophysiological mechanisms underlying the understanding and imitation of action. Nat Rev Neurosci 2001;2: 661–670.
72 Pike FH: An apology for yawning. J Hered 1916;7: 447–449.
73 Hughlings Jackson J: Yawning. Lancet 1905;165:174.
74 Von Economo C: Encephalitis lethargica and its sequelae and treatment. London, Oxford Medical Publications, 1931.
75 Sicard JA, Paraff A: Fou rire syncopal et bâillements au cours de l'encéphalite épidémique. Bull Mem Soc Med Hop Paris 1921;45:232–233.
76 Levy G: Contribution à l'étude des manifestations tardives de l'encéphalite épidémique. Paris, Vigot, 1922.
77 Hall A: Epidemic Encephalitis. Bristol, John Wright and Sons, 1924.
78 Jelliffe SE: Postencephalitic Respiratory Disorders. New York, Nervous and Mental Disease Publishing Company, 1927.
79 De Saussure R: Discussion sur l'étiologie d'un tic survenu quinze mois après une encéphalite léthargique atypique. Arch Suisse Neurol Psychiatrie 1923;12:292–317.
80 Guillin G, Mollaret P: Les séquelles de l'encéphalite épidémique. Paris, Doin, 1932.
81 Claparède E: Pourquoi bâille-t-on? Genève, Institut JJ Rousseau, L'éducateur 1924;60:65–70.
82 Dumpert V: Zur Kenntnis des Wesens und der physiologischen Bedeutung des Gähnens. J Psychol Neurol 1921;27:82–95.
83 Delmas-Marsallet P: Le signe du bâillement dans les lésions du cerveau frontal. Otoneuroophtalmologie 1937;15:183.
84 Heusner AP: Yawning and associated phenomena. Physiol Rev 1946;25:156–168.
85 Barbizet J: Yawning. J Neurol Neurosurg Psychiat 1958;21:203–209.
86 Furtado D: Consideraçoes sobre o bocejo (a proposito de um caso clinico). Gaz Med Port 1949;1:983–989.
87 Montagu A: On yawning. JAMA 1962;732:152.
88 Boudouresque J, Pache R, Khalil R: Troubles réflexes viscéraux. EMC fev 1965:17102D10.
89 Ferrari W, Gessa, GL, Vargiu L: Behavioral effects induced by intracisternally injected ACTH and MSH. Ann NY Acad Sci 1963;104:330.
90 Urba-Holmgren R, Gonzalez RM, Holmgren B: Is yawning a cholinergic response? Nature 1977;267: 261–262.
91 Provine RR, Tate BC, Gelmacher LL: Yawning : no effects of 3–5% CO_2, 100% O_2 and exercise. Behav Neural Biol 1987;48:382–393.
92 Baenninger R, Binkley S, Baenninger M: Field observations of yawning and activity in humans. Physiol Behav 1996;59:421–425.
93 Deputte BL, Johnson J, Hempel M, Scheffler G: Behavioral effects of an antiandrogen in adult male rhesus macaques (*Macaca mulatta*). Horm Behav 1994;28:155–164.
94 Troisi A, Aureli F, Schino G, et al: The influence of age, sex, rank on yawning behavior in two species of macaques. Ethology 1990;86:303–313.

Dr. Olivier Walusinski
20 rue de Chartres
FR–28160 Brou (France)
Tel. +33 2 37 47 07 77, Fax +33 2 37 47 19 07
E-Mail walusinski@baillement.com

Walusinski O (ed): The Mystery of Yawning in Physiology and Disease.
Front Neurol Neurosci. Basel, Karger, 2010, vol 28, pp 22–25

Popular Knowledge and Beliefs

Olivier Walusinski

General Practice, Brou, France

Abstract

Although few things are as common as yawning, it has traditionally held little interest for researchers and enquiring minds of all disciplines. Yawning is a recognized behavior in almost all vertebrates, present throughout life, which often procures a sense of well-being for the yawner.

Modern science is still searching for a complete explanation of the mechanisms and purpose of yawning, with debate about its usefulness as a stimulatory mechanism still ongoing. In this paper, we offer an overview of the popular beliefs and myths seen within Arabic, Western and Indian cultures.

Since antiquity, yawning has held as little interest for philosophers, psychologists and physiologists as it has for teachers, moralists and physicians. And yet, few things are as common as yawning. Everyone yawns 5–10 times a day. Yawning is a recognized behavior in almost all vertebrates, from birds to humans; one which starts in the womb and continues until death. Although yawning often procures a sense of well-being for the yawner, attempting to mask this behavior is common practice worldwide.

Modern neuroscience is still looking for a complete explanation of the intimate mechanisms of yawning. Moreover, its exact physiological purpose remains a subject of debate: some see yawning as a mechanism for stimulating wakefulness [1], while others contest this view and instead link yawing to sleepiness, but do not provide evidence for an arousing effect of yawning [2].

In this paper, we offer a broad-based cultural overview of the related conceptions and myths through a comparison of the popular views within Arabic, Western and Indian cultures.

Arab Countries

In 1921, Pierre Saintyves surveyed cultural beliefs related to the meaning of yawning. According to Saintyves, Islam sees yawning as a sign of Satan entering the body, and sneezing as a sign of his leaving the body. Assas-bou-Malek and others all date this opinion back to the Prophet [3]:

> The Prophet said that Satan endeavors to distract the faithful in prayer. This is Allah's way of testing them. One way Satan distracts the faithful is by dominating their thoughts, infiltrating their minds during prayer. Another way is by making them yawn to divert attention away from their prayers. The Prophet told us that yawning is prompted by Satan and gave us the order to avoid it whenever possible. When it becomes inevitable, we must close our mouth with our hand.

We recently came across this question on a website:

> I am a 22-year-old devout practising Muslim with a problem I hope to overcome with Allah's help and your advice. As soon as I begin my prayers, I start yawning involuntarily. And this continues even when I recite the Throne Verse. I really don't know why I'm yawning dozens of times, over and over, during a single prayer. I hope you can shed some light on my problem.

Saintyves also writes: 'According to Ibn Battal, attributing yawning to Satan means he wants us to yawn and takes pleasure in it; he enjoys this disfiguring behavior because it makes men look ridiculous.' As to putting a hand over the mouth, this gesture applies when the mouth is already open, as well as when it is stiffly closed, 'because Satan enters …'. Instead of the hand, a piece of clothing or any other object may be used. The fear of Satan entering the body is linked to the fear of possession, which explains why this gesture is demanded of the faithful during prayer [4]. W. Seuntjens call this idea the demonic rationale of yawning etiquette [5]. Moroccans would place their hand in front of their gaping mouth because otherwise, it was believed, the devil would urinate into their mouth.

India

In India, 'bhuts' (spirits) are believed to prefer entering the body through the mouth. Yawning is therefore dangerous because it entails two kinds of risks: either bhuts penetrate the body through the throat, or a part of the soul might escape. Since it would be very difficult to recapture, the recommended practice is to put a hand in front of one's mouth and say 'Narayan!' ('good God!'), or snap one's fingers to scare the bad spirit away [3].

In ancient Mayan civilization, yawning was thought to indicate subconscious sexual desires. In the same way, W. Seuntjens hypothesized that yawning has an erotic side. He found that both the 'yawn' and the 'stretch' of the stretch-yawn syndrome are semantically and etymologically associated with 'desire' and 'longing'. In several proverbs and sayings, yawning, and especially contagious yawning, is interpreted as a clue of something more than just sympathy, i.e. of being in love. Yawning was both linked with acedia-boredom and with luxuria (lechery) and passion. As a non-verbal behavior, the yawn was found to figure in the courtship process. The fact that this is not just a recent or Western phenomenon has been illustrated by passages from ancient Indian literature [6].

Europe

Around 590 AD, during the time of Pope Gregory the Great, a bubonic plague epidemic raged through Europe, decimating the population and inspiring numerous superstitions [7]:

> Yawning was fatal then, and the habit of signing the cross in front of the mouth originated during the times of the plague … There was a plague they called inguinal, because a bubo appeared in the groins, causing men to die suddenly in the streets, in their houses, at play, during a meal. Their souls left their bodies when they sneezed or yawned. This is why we said 'God bless you' to those who sneezed. Those who yawned made the sign of the cross over their mouths.

Even the skeptical Michel de Montaigne made the sign of the cross before his mouth while yawning, showing the power surrounding this belief. In Austria, when a yawning baby was not able to perform the sign of the cross, an older person would perform this gesture in front of the infant's mouth in order to prevent illness and bad luck.

It is possible that the love of perfumes in the royal European courts in the 17th and 18th centuries had its origins in the necessity to conceal poor body hygiene. Placing one's hand in front of the mouth during yawning was helpful in hiding appalling oral conditions and reducing the expiration of nauseating odors. In a 2004 editorial for the *British Medical Journal*, G. Dunea was surprised to see medical students yawning frequently as they waited for their lecturer; moreover, 67.5% of the time they did not cover their mouths with their hands. He suggested this allowed students to avoid bacterial contamination of their palms, ironically adding that it is undoubtedly better to let others marvel at your tonsils than to risk injuring your elbow! [8].

Yawing in Medicine

In his treatise on wind, *De flatibus liber*, Hippocrates noted that 'the continual yawning of apoplectics proves that air is the cause of apoplexies', thereby confirming his theory that 'wind is the cause of all diseases' [9]. In 1739, Hermann Boerhaave, in his *Praelectiones academicae*, explained that 'yawning and pandiculation favor the suitable distribution of spiritus in all the muscles and unblock the vessels of which sleep or rest may have slowed the functions', and that their action fights 'against the excessive pre-eminence of the flexor muscles and returns everything to its place' [10]. In his 1755 book, *De perspiratione insensibii*, Johan de Gorter was the first to suggest that yawning accelerates blood flow, supposedly to improve the oxygenation of the brain, in response to cerebral anemia [11]. Well into the 20th century, there were regular references to this notion, even though it had never been demonstrated. Even someone as knowledgeable and inquisitive as J.M. Charcot repeated this maxim without any critical analysis in his *Leçons du Mardi à la Salpêtrière* in 1888 [12]. The inaccuracy of this hypothesis was formally shown by Provine et al. [13] in 1987. They had their subjects inhale air with higher than normal levels of CO_2 (3–5 vs. <0.5%). In response, the subjects' breathing rates increased, but they did not yawn. Likewise, when the subjects inhaled pure oxygen, there was no inhibition of spontaneous yawning at normal rates. Hence, yawning is not a physiological reflex to improve cerebral oxygenation.

References

1 Askenazy JJ: Yawing: an arousal defense reflex? J Psychol 1989;123:609–621.
2 Guggisberg AG, Mathis J, Herrniann US, Hess CW: The fictional relationship between yawning and vigilance. Behav Brain Res 2007;179:159–166.
3 Saintyves P: L'éternuement et le bâillement dans la magie, l'ethnographie et le folklore médical. Paris, Emile Nourry, 1921.
4 El Bokhâri: Les traditions islamiques (traduites de l'arabe avec notes et index par O. Houdas et W. Marçais). Paris, Imprimerie Nationale, vol W, 211213, pp 1903–1914.
5 Seuntjens W: On yawning or the hidden sexuality of the human yawn; thesis, Amsterdam, Vrije University, 2004, p 491.
6 Vâtsyâyana M: Kâmasûtra (translation from Sanskrit: Doniger W, Kakar S). Paris, Le Seuil, 2007, p 430.
7 Le Camus A: La médecine pratique rendue plus simple, plus sûre et plus méthodique. Paris, Gagneau Lib., 1769, p 477.
8 Dunea G: On covering one's mouth (when yawning). BMJ 2004;328:963.
9 Hippocrate: Open omnia. Anuce Foes. Frankfurt am Main, Wechel héritiers d'André 1595, p 379. www.bium.univ-pariss.fr/histmed/medica.htm.
10 Boerhaave H: Praelectiones academicae in proprias institutiones rei medicae. Gottingae, A. Vandenhoeck Imp., 1741–1745, vol 4.
11 de Gorter J: De perspiratione insensibii. Patavii, J. Manfrè, 1755, p 328.
12 Charcot JM: Leçons du lardi à La Salpêtrière. Paris, Bureaux du Progrès Médical et Delahaye A, 1887.
13 Provine RR, Tate BC, Geldmacher LL: Yawning: no effect of 3–5% CO_2, 100% O_2, and exercise. Behav Neural Biol 1987;48:382–393.

Dr. Olivier Walusinski
20 rue de Chartres
FR–28160 Brou (France)
Tel. +33 2 37 47 07 77, Fax +33 2 37 47 19 07
E-Mail walusinski@baillement.com

Walusinski O (ed): The Mystery of Yawning in Physiology and Disease.
Front Neurol Neurosci. Basel, Karger, 2010, vol 28, pp 26–31

Yawning throughout Life

F. Giganti · P. Salzarulo

Department of Psychology, University of Florence, Florence, Italy

Abstract

Yawning is a behavior that begins in the first stages of life. It has not only been observed in infants and in newborns, but also in fetuses of 12–14 weeks' gestational age. Yawning frequency changes over the life span. In preterm infants, the number of yawns decreases between 31 and 40 weeks' postconceptional age, mainly during the day. In this period of life, yawning is an isolated behavior rarely occurring in bursts, and its frequency is quite low with respect to adults. The incidence of yawning seems to increase when children attend elementary school, whereas this is reduced in the elderly. Aged people yawn less than younger ones, mainly during morning and mid-afternoon. In adults, the time course of yawning is associated with the time course of sleepiness, except upon awakening when the high frequency of yawns is not associated with high sleepiness. In adults, yawning frequency increases in the early morning and in the late evening, whereas at the earliest stages of development (fetuses and preterm infants) yawning does not show diurnal variations. Yawning seems to be involved in the modulation of arousal process across the whole life span. In preterm infants, yawning is often followed by motor activation and it is more common during waking than sleep; in adults, yawning occurs mainly at sleep onset and upon awakening.

Yawning is a mysterious behavior that can assume different meanings. Spontaneous yawning is present in humans from the early stages of development, and apparently linked to sleep-wake transitions and the modulation of arousal processes. However, yawning is also contagious, i.e. it can be elicited by viewing or hearing other people yawning. During development, this 'contagious' form of yawning is observed later than the 'spontaneous' yawn.

In this chapter, the frequency and time course changes of spontaneous yawning across the life span will be examined, taking into account hypotheses about its role and function. In addition, contagious yawning will be examined in order to better understand the nature of spontaneous and contagious yawning and to clarify underlying differences between them.

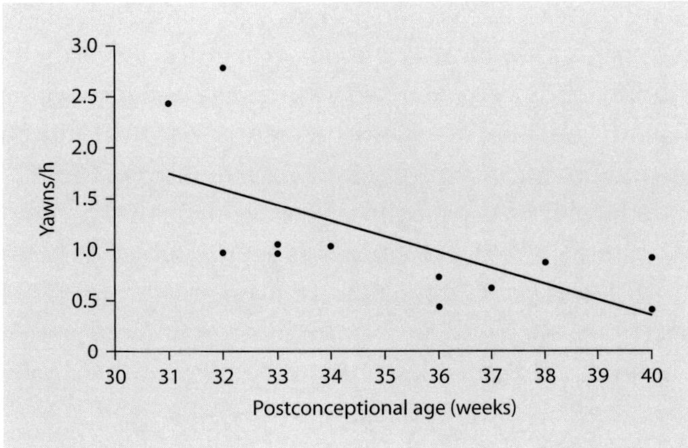

Fig. 1. Number of yawns per hour (across the 24-hour period) in preterm and near-term infants. Reproduced with kind permission [4].

Features and Frequency of Yawning

The presence of yawning was initially observed in fetuses between 12 and 14 weeks' gestational age [1]; this was recently confirmed by Walusinki [2].

Yawning has also recently been described in preterm infants during the final weeks before term age [3, 4]. In this period of life, the frequency of yawns is higher than that reported in adults (approx. 25 vs. 7–8/24 h) [5]. It is worth pointing out that in babies yawning is often an isolated event not yet organized into consistent bursts and rarely accompanied by the stretching seen in adults [3, 4]. This fits with the developmental trend of other physiological and behavioral activities, e.g. eye movements during sleep [6, 7], which are isolated early in life and have not yet been organized into the bursts seen in adults.

During the last weeks before term age, yawning can occur not only in the waking state, but also during drowsiness and (less frequently) in active sleep; it is very rarely observed in quiet sleep [3, 4]. In preterm infants, the presence of yawns is associated with motor activity in the waking state of infants, whereas low levels of activity seem to discourage yawning [4]. A fine-grained analysis investigating the temporal relationship between yawning and motor activation in the infant is necessary to support the hypothesis of the activation role of yawning suggested by many authors in adults [8–11].

The frequency of yawns changes across the life span. Although in the fetus the incidence of yawns does not change between 20 and 36 weeks' gestational age [12], in preterm infants the frequency during the 24-week period decreases significantly between 31 and 40 weeks' gestational age (fig. 1), mainly during the daytime [4]. This reduction occurs at the same time of the day as the waking episode duration increases [13], supporting the hypothesis that 'the improvement in wake stability during the diurnal period may reflect the decreased need of yawning to support or stabilize the arousal level' [4, p. 646].

In infants observed after term age, yawning usually occurs before sleep onset as a 'signal' of sleepiness or sleep proximity. Nevertheless, many sleep episodes start without being preceded by yawning and the interval between yawns and sleep onset is quite variable [14]. Unfortunately, Wolff [14] did not present data on changes in yawning frequency during the first 6 months of life.

At later ages, when children attend elementary school, yawning frequency seems to increase with respect to previous ages. Koch et al. [15] found an increase in yawning in kindergarten children, and an even greater increase in children attending the first year of primary school (5 times more than in kindergarten children). More recently, Chouard and Bigot-Massoni [16] confirmed the significant increase in yawning frequency when children learn to write and to read.

Studies on sleep-wake rhythms in the adolescent reported an increase in sleepiness around the middle of the day [17]. Taking into account the increase in sleepiness at that time [18] and the strong relationship between yawning and sleepiness widely documented by several researches [5, 8, 19, 20], we can put forward the hypothesis that the rise in sleepiness could be accompanied by an increase in yawning frequency.

As previously mentioned, the frequency in the adult is about 7–8/24 h, with a large difference between individuals (0–30/24 h). An explanation of the large inter-individual differences comes from studies comparing different typologies of sleeper. The daily number of yawns tends to be higher in evening types compared to morning types [21], and in long sleepers compared to short sleepers [unpubl. data].

In the elderly, the frequency of yawning seems to be reduced compared to young adults [22]. This reduction has been clearly confirmed by a recent study [23], which also showed that the decrease in yawning is mainly present in the morning and mid-afternoon.

Time Course of Yawning

The time course of yawning differs as a function of age [5]. In adults, the frequency of yawning increases in the early morning and late evening [8, 11], i.e. following awakening and preceding sleep onset [5, 19] when sleepiness is high.

In adults, the time course of yawning is associated with the time course of sleepiness, although there is an exception upon waking where elderly adults show no association between the frequency of yawning and the sleepiness level [23]. These data suggest that sleepiness level and sleep episode proximity could affect yawning production separately.

Differently with respect to adults who show a peak in the early morning and in the evening, in preterm and near term infants yawning is uniformly distributed over the 24-hour period [4]. The reason is that while the relationship between yawning and sleep-wake transition (well-known in adults [19]) is already established in neonates

[14] and possibly in preterm infants, at very early ages there are several sleep and wake episodes over 24 h. As a result, the increase in the frequency of yawning at the daytime wake-sleep transitions leads to a flattening of the curve. The characteristic time course of yawning (a peak after awakening and another peak late in the evening) is progressively built up and does not appear until the fourth year, when a monophasic sleep-wake rhythm has been established and children usually stop sleeping during the day [24]. Thus, morning and evening peaks of yawning become linked to the establishment of the circadian sleep-wake rhythm.

Yawning and Arousal Processes

In the young adults, yawning is linked to a low level of vigilance and its production usually increases before and after a sleep episode when sleepiness is high [19] and when subjects are bored or engaged in repetitive and monotonous activities [25]. These results led to the view of yawning as a way of enhancing arousal levels [5, 8]. Evidence for this hypothesis comes from studies that found an increase in motility [5] and brain activation [26, 27] after yawning. Nevertheless, some authors disagree with this argument as they could not find an arousing effect on the brain (measured by electroencephalogram recordings) or the autonomic nervous system (measured by hearth rate variability) in patients with excessive sleepiness [28].

Contagious Yawning

Viewing or listening to somebody else yawning may evoke yawning in the observer/listener [20]. In young adults, yawning is contagious in 55% of subjects within 5 min; even thinking about yawning can induce it in 88% of subjects within 30 min [11]. This means that yawning is not only a 'spontaneous behavior' which is related to the regulation of vigilance levels, but also a 'response' to environmental conditions (both social and physical). How the latter could be facilitated by the former? Surprisingly a preliminary study by our group [unpubl. data] showed that the contagious effect of yawning also occurs when subjects are not prone to spontaneous yawning, suggesting that different factors could be involved in the two kinds of yawning. This result is in agreement with a developmental trend which shows an asynchrony between the ages at which spontaneous and contagious yawing are first observed. In fact, the contagious form is only observed from 4–5 years of age onwards [29]. This time lag between the emergence of the two kinds of yawning leads one to suspect they have different underlying factors.

At later ages, the percentage of children showing contagious yawning is even higher [30] than those reported by Provine [11] in young adults. Indeed 70% of 12-year-old children yawn when viewing others yawning (vs. 55% of adult subjects).

The difference between children and adults is probably due to the lower social inhibition of yawning in children than in young adults.

In summary, we have shown that during the first stages of development only spontaneous yawning is present, at a relatively low frequency; in the young adults, this decreases, and even more so in the elderly. Furthermore, the daily distribution of spontaneous yawning changes: in preterm infants yawning does not show diurnal variation, whereas in young adults and the elderly there is an increase in the early morning and in the late evening, respectively, after and before the main sleep episode. In contrast, the link between spontaneous yawning and the modulation of vigilance levels seems to be maintained across the whole life span. At very early ages, yawning is present during drowsiness and the waking state, possibly associated with the effort required to remain awake; in young adults and the elderly, these occur mainly at sleep onset and upon awakening, when the sleepiness level is high.

Contagious yawning occurs later in life than the spontaneous yawning. In addition, the contagious effect of yawning seems to be independent of the propensity to spontaneously yawn. This result and the phase shift between the emergence of the two kinds of yawning support the hypothesis that they have different underlying factors.

References

1 de Vries JIP, Visser GHA, Prechtl HFR: The emergence of fetal behavior. I. Qualitative aspects. Early Hum Dev 1982;7:301–322.

2 Walusinski O, Kurjak A, Andonotopo W, Azumendi G: Fetal yawning assessed by 3D and 4D sonography. Ultrasound Rev Obstet Gynecol 2005;5:210–217.

3 Giganti F, Hayes MJ, Akilesh MR, Salzarulo P: Yawning and behavioral states in premature infants. Dev Psychobiol 2002;41:289–296.

4 Giganti F, Hayes M, Cioni G, Salzarulo P: Yawning frequency and distribution in preterm and near term infants assessed throughout 24-h recordings. Infant Behav Dev 2007;30:641–647.

5 Baenninger R, Binkley S, Baenninger M: Field observations of yawning and activity in humans. Physiol Behav 1996;59:421–425.

6 Birnholz JC: The development of human fetal eye-movement patterns. Science 1981;213:679–681.

7 Ktonas PY, Bes F, Rigoard MT, Wong C, Mallart R, Salzarulo P: Developmental changes in the clustering pattern of sleep rapid eye movement activity during the first year of life: a Markov-process approach. Electroenceph Clin Neurophysiol 1990; 75:136–140.

8 Baenninger R: On yawning and its functions. Psychon B Rev 1997;4:198–207.

9 Daquin G, Micallef J, Blin O: Yawning. Sleep Med Rev 2001;5:299–312.

10 Walusinski O, Deputte BL: Le baillement: Phylogenese, ethologie, nosogenie. Rev Neurol 2004; 160:1011–1021.

11 Provine RR: Yawning. Am Sci 2005;93:532–539.

12 Roodenburg PJ, Wladimiroff JW, van Es A, Prechtl HFR: Classification and quantitative aspects of fetal movements during the second half of normal pregnancy. Early Hum Dev 1991;25:19–35.

13 Giganti F, Ficca G, Cioni G, Salzarulo P: Spontaneous awakenings in preterm and term infants assessed throughout 24-hour video-recordings. Early Hum Dev 2006;82:435–440.

14 Wolff PH: The Development of Behavioral States and the Expressions of Emotions in Early Infancy. Chicago, University Chicago Press, 1987.

15 Koch P, Montagner H, Soussignan R : Variation of behavioural and physiological variables in children attending kindergarten and primary school. Chronobiol Int 1987;4:525–535.

16 Chouard CH, Bigot-Massoni D: Mécanismes et rôle physiologique du bâillement. Ann Otolaryngol Chir Cervicofac 1990;107:145–153.
17 Palm L, Persson E, Elmquist D, Blennow G: Sleep and wakefulness in normal and preadolescent children. Sleep 1989;12:299–308.
18 Carskadon MA: Patterns of sleep and sleepiness in adolescent. Pediatrician 1990;17:5–12.
19 Provine RR, Hamernik HB, Curchack BB: Yawning: relation to sleeping and stretching in humans. Ethology 1987;76:152–160.
20 Provine RR: Yawning as a stereotyped action pattern and releasing stimulus. Ethology 1986;72:109–122.
21 Zilli I, Giganti F, Salzarulo P: Yawning in morning and evening types. Physiol Behav 2007;91:218–222.
22 Walusinski O: Le bâillement: naissance, vie et sénescence. Psychol Neuropsychiatr Vieill 2006;4:39–46.
23 Zilli I, Giganti F, Uga V: Yawning and subjective sleepiness in the elderly. J Sleep Res 2008;17:303–308.
24 Acebo C, Sadeh A, Seifer R, Tzischinsky O, Hafer A, Carskadon MA: Sleep/wake patterns derived from activity monitoring and maternal report for healthy 1- to 5-year-old children. Sleep 2005;28:1568–1577.
25 Provine RR, Hamernik HB: Yawning: effects of stimulus interest. B Psychonomic Soc 1986;24:437–438.
26 Karasawa J, Kuriyama Y, Kuro M, Kikuchi H, Sawada T, Mitsugi T: Monitoring system of cerebral blood flow and cerebral metabolism: relationship between internal jugular oxygen tension and cerebral blood flow. Brain Nerve 1982;34:239–245.
27 Kasuya Y, Murakami T, Oshima T, Dohi S: Does yawning represent a transient arousal-shift during intravenous induction of general anesthesia? Anesth Analg 2005;100:382–384.
28 Guggisberg AG, Mathis J, Herrmann US, Hess CW: The functional relationship between yawning and vigilance. Behav Brain Res 2007;179:159–166.
29 Anderson JR, Meno P: Psychological influences on yawning in children. Curr Psychol Lett 2003;11. http://cpl.revues.org/document390.html.
30 Giganti F, Ziello M: Contagious and spontaneous yawning in autistic and typically developing children. Curr Psychol Lett 2009;25. http://cpl.revues.org/index4810.html.

Fiorenza Giganti
Department of Psychology, University of Florence
Via di San Salvi 12, Complesso di San Salvi, Padiglione 26
IT–50135 Florence (Italy)
Tel. +39 055 6237853, Fax +39 055 6236047, E-Mail fiorenza.giganti@unifi.it

Walusinski O (ed): The Mystery of Yawning in Physiology and Disease.
Front Neurol Neurosci. Basel, Karger, 2010, vol 28, pp 32–41

Fetal Yawning

Olivier Walusinski

General Practice, Brou, France

Abstract

Fetal neurobehavioral patterns have been considered as indicators of nervous system development. Moreover, the capacity of 4-dimensional sonography to evaluate complex facial expressions allows recognition of common behaviors with which one can appreciate the prenatal functional development of the central nervous system. Using yawning as an example, we review this interpretation on the basis of knowledge derived from phylogeny and ontogeny. As a flip-flop switch, the reciprocal interactions between sleep- and wake-promoting brain regions allow the emergence of distinct states of arousal. By its ontogenic links with REM sleep, yawning appears to be a behavior which causes arousal reinforcement through the powerful stretching and the neuromuscular connections induced. Yawning indicates a harmonious progress in the development of both the brainstem and the peripheral neuromuscular function, testifying to the induction of an ultradian rhythm of vigilance. The lack of fetal yawn, frequently associated with lack of swallowing (associated or not with retrognathia), may be a key to predicting brainstem dysfunction after birth.

General movements are part of the repertoire of spontaneous movement, and are present from early fetal life. Prior to the 1970s, self-perception by mothers was the only testimony of this fetal motor activity. The advent of ultrasound technology in the 1970s enabled live unobtrusive observations of fetal behaviors in humans, vastly increasing our knowledge of many other types of more subtle motor activity (swallowing, respiratory movements, smiling, hiccups) and thus human fetal development. Our understanding of the developmental order and sequence of fetal behavior increased substantially, leading to a greater appreciation of embryologic and developmental anatomy. The introduction of 4-dimensional ultrasound (4D-US) has led to very important conclusions concerning fetal behavior milestones [1]. The development of oral sensorimotor function and swallowing (essential for survival) from the fetal period through early infancy indicates normal or abnormal neurobehavioral development. While the appreciation of these functions takes a long time, another daily behavior will can be detected: yawning [2]. Curiously, little data has been published over the last 25 years, since the following was written: 'yawning is a universally well known, but poorly understood' [3] or 'a rudimentary reflex' and 'appears to have at best an obscure purpose, if any' [4]. Although remarkably little interest has been paid to yawning in research (despite the fact it is an everyday phenomenon), we will discuss the meaning of this behavior and how its characterization can enhance neurobehavioral understanding.

First however, it must be specified that human research on prenatal programming of behavior is intrinsically correlational, never manipulatively experimental, and frequently based upon homologies with others vertebrates.

A popular saying states that 'the organ generates the function'. However, embryology instructs us that body movement in a fetus is required for maturation of motor function and is involved in the development of other organs, such as the lung. Furthermore, body movement indicates an harmonious progression in the development of both the central motor system and peripheral neuromuscular function [5]. All the movements that a newborn is able to produce originate during the fetal life and are performed throughout the life span. Behaviors observed in utero – including breathing, yawning and others – are a part of the continuum of activity shown in a newborn infant and undergo neuromuscular rewiring. The onset and developmental course of fetal motility have been studied since ultrasound technology appeared; however, the evaluation of facial expressions was impossible using real-time 2D-US. In particular, it was the capacity of 4D-US to evaluate complex facial expressions that allowed recognition of yawning [2, 6, 7].

What Is a Yawn?

de Vries et al. [8] have proposed a classification of fetal movement patterns studied longitudinally: the first movement is observable during the 7th postconceptional week; generalized trunk and limb movements by the 9th week; movements of the fetal jaw and face observed around the 11th week. Yawning is recognized as one of the movement patterns consistently present from the end of the first trimester until delivery.

A yawn is a paroxysmic cycle characterized by a standard cascade of movements over a 5- to 10-second period. The 4D-US differentiates this typical development: the fetal mouth, previously closed, opens widely for 4–6 s with simultaneous retraction of the tongue, followed by a quick closure, and usually combined with retroflexion of the head and sometimes elevation of the arms (pandiculation) [9]. This harmonious sequence is markedly different than a brief swallowing episode. Using a color Doppler technique, it is possible to observe the flow of amniotic fluid through the fetal mouth, oropharynx, pharynx and trachea to the lungs [10]. This movement pattern is non-repetitive in the fetus, contrarily to adults. Yawning appears to be clearly not just a matter of opening one's mouth, but a generalized stretching of muscles, especially those of the respiratory tract (diaphragm, intercostals), face and neck. Thus, it can be inferred that yawning is a part of the generalized stretch with which it is generally accompanied [11].

Embryology and Mechanisms

In 1973, T. Dobzhansky remarked: 'nothing in biology makes sense except in the light of evolution.' Ernst von Haeckel (1834–1919) stated that: 'ontogenesis is a brief and rapid recapitulation of phylogenesis, determined by the physiological functions of heredity (generation) and adaptation (maintenance).' The truth of these quotations is illustrated by yawning. Indeed, the ultrasound investigation reveals an ontogenic onset between 12 and 15 weeks of gestation [2]. Indeed, yawning is a phylogenetically old and stereotyped phenomena that occurs in a huge variety of species, from reptiles and fish to birds and mammals. Its survival without evolutionary variations postulates a particular importance in terms of developmental need [9]. The strong muscular contraction that represents a yawn has a metabolically expensive cost. If we agree with the terms of the Darwin's evolutionary propositions, the cost in brain activity must be outweighed by the advantages gained in terms of developmental fitness. Thus, a structural hypothesis suggests an activation in the synthesis of neurotrophins which leads to a cascade of both new synapse formation or recruitment and activation through the diencephalon, brainstem and spinal cord. The phenomenon of activity-dependent development has been clearly shown to be one mechanism by which early sensory or motor experience can affect the course of neural development. Activity-dependent development may be a ubiquitous process in brain maturation by which activity in one brain region can influence the developmental course of other regions [12].

A wealth of data has been accumulated on genes that are expressed in the embryo and govern the hindbrain segmentation. Hox homeobox genes form 4 conserved clusters encoding transcription factors that orchestrate ontogenesis along the rostro-caudal axis of the body, including hindbrain segmentation and limb formation. The facial bone structure and the brain differentiate from a common embryonic structure, the ectoblast. The cephalic pole comprises an original embryological encephalo-facial and encephalo-cervical segmentation with a strict topographical correspondence: the naso-frontal and premaxillary structures are joined to the forebrain; the maxillo-mandibular and anterior cervical structures are joined to the brainstem and its nerves [13–15]. The human brainstem is fashioned around the 6th–7th week of gestation and matures in a caudal to rostral arc, thereby forming the medulla, pons and midbrain. The medulla mediates arousal, breathing, heart rate, and gross movements of the body and head, and medullary functions appear prior to those of the pons, which precede those of the midbrain [16]. The ability to produce motor behavior generated centrally and linked to arousal and respiratory function is a property of the brainstem reticular formation, which has been remarkably conserved during the phylogeny of vertebrates including agnathans, fishes, amphibians, reptiles and birds. Therefore, conservative developmental mechanisms orchestrating the organogenesis of the brainstem in all vertebrates are probably crucial for arousal and breathing [17]. At the beginning of the 3rd month, the embryo becomes a fetus with the occurrence of the first oral and pharyngeal motor sequences under the control of the neurological development of the brainstem, such as suction-deglutition and yawning activity. Therefore, suction and yawning have the same embryological origin, which shows the importance of the brainstem in the neurophysiological development of the oropharyngeal activity coordinated with the respiratory, cardiac and digestive regulations that have the same neuroanatomical localization. Its occurrence marks the developmental stage when the brainstem is already individualized and the pituitary gland has become functional, whereas the extension of the temporal and frontal neocortex takes up to 22–24 weeks to reach completion [18–20]. Movements of the tongue or jaw assist the development of the palate by promoting horizontal elevation of vertically orientated palatal shelves. Activity of neck and tongue muscles are always accompanied by mouth-tongue movement [21]. The relationship or connection between the neural network of mouth-tongue movement and respiratory activities are not perfectly understood. It seems that information about central respiratory and locomotor rhythms, necessary for cerebellum control of the coordination between respiration and locomotion, converges at the level of the lateral reticular nucleus [22]. It is probable that the explanation for craniofacial congenital developmental abnormalities, which ultrasound investigation helps to reveal, lies here. As the saying goes: 'the face predicts the brain.'

Why Does Yawning Share a Link with Arousal?

The phylogenetic appearance of sleep suggests that the nocturnal rest of poikilotherms most probably becomes in mammals a form of REM sleep or paradoxical sleep, which is characterized by peripheral muscular atonia originating in the dorsal part of the brainstem, rostral to the pons [23].

Based on numerous studies of fetuses and infants in a variety of mammalian species, it is widely believed that the earliest form of sleep is properly characterized as active sleep, which is an immature form of REM sleep and preponderant at birth. Accordingly, it is thought that quiet sleep, an immature form of slow-wave sleep, emerges as the predominance of REM sleep diminishes during ontogeny [24].

In early intrauterine life, a diffuse collection of phasic and cyclic motor events occur, and these gradually coalesce. For the fetus, sleep and wakefulness are reliably characterized, respectively, by periods of myoclonic twitching expressed against a background of muscle atonia and high-amplitude behaviors (e.g. locomotion or stretching-yawning) expressed against a background of high muscle tone. Movements of the limbs, such as stretching, yawning and kicking, are typically considered to indicate periods of wakefulness. Periods of twitching are almost always followed by the abrupt onset of high-amplitude awake behaviors, thus completing the cycle. Although myoclonic twitching during active sleep in infants is more prevalent and more intense than that seen during REM sleep in adults, its similarities to adult behavior and its linkage to periods of atonia suggest developmental continuity between the infant and adult sleep states. The maturation of the central nervous system, based on the myelinization, starts in the spinal cord then proceeds to the brainstem and forebrain. So, paradoxical sleep mechanisms located in the brainstem are the first to mature and the only ones to function. Then, the slow-wave sleep and waking structures become mature. Namely, the widespread control of neuronal activity exerted by specific REM sleep processes help to direct brain maturation through activity-dependent developmental mechanisms. It may be inferred that REM sleep (and possibly yawning) directs the course of brain maturation in early life through the control of neural activity [25, 26].

Behavioral pattern continuity from prenatal to postnatal life shows a strict parallelism between the ontogeny of REM sleep and yawning. Basically, REM sleep in the human declines from 50% of total sleep time (8 h) and a frequency of 30–50 yawns per day in the newborn to 15% of total sleep time (1 h) and less than 20 yawns per day in the adult. This decrease takes place mainly between birth and the end of puberty [27].

The emergence of distinct states is followed by dramatic changes in the amount, duration and cyclicity of rest and activity. An ultradian rhythm may be seen: in a period of 50–60 minutes there appears to be an alternation of moments characterized by motor activity and moments characterized by rest, as in the newborn [28]. Each period of rest switches over to a period of activity by a yawn. Thus, a periodicity of 1–2 yawns per hour can be noticed. Yawning appears 2 weeks before discernable sleep-wake states, and its expression gradually becomes linked. No changes in the incidence of yawns between 20 and 36 weeks of gestational age were observed in the fetus by P.J. Roodenburg [29]. In full-term infants, yawns are frequently observed on the first day of life. The embryo and the fetus are exposed to 24-hour periodicity in mothers' parameters of the circadian cycle that may play a role in the normal development of the fetus pacemaker. No data are available on how fetal yawning links up fetal rhythm with maternal rhythm.

C. Saper [30] proposed a model for reciprocal interactions between sleep- and wake-promoting brain regions, which produces a flip-flop switch. This model could explain the rapid transitions from awaking in sleep and from REM sleep to awaking. It is a survival necessity to ensure a repairing sleep while having the capacity to flee a predator (arousal). The transition is controlled by integrative autonomic structures that encompass regulated changes occurring in anticipation of the event. Yawning (a stretch syndrome) can be seen as a behavior for testing this switch/transition, like a reinforcement of muscle tone. Awakening is controlled by around 4 different and redundant circuits mainly located in the reticular formation of the pons (adrenergic), the peduncle (dopaminergic), the hypothalamus (histaminergic) and the Meynert basifrontal region (cholinergic). The permissive networks controlling awakening must be tonically reinforced by the hypocretin system originating in the lateral hypothalamus. Next, the neuron's activation of the ventrolateral preoptic nucleus (VLPO) is correlated with the amount of sleep. The powerful muscular contraction caused by yawning releases arousal by activation of the reticular formation (locus coeruleus), to which the cranial nerves send retro-projections. On becoming aware, the yawning and stretching reverse the muscular atonia which characterizes REM sleep. When the pressure of sleep increases, it is supposed that the firing of the GABA and galanin VLPO neurons reduce the muscular tone of antigravitational muscles, notably those of the neck and masseters. Thus, yawning seems to be averse to this pressure. F. Giganti et al. [32] observed yawning in premature infants in all behavioral states, except during quiet sleep, and viewed it as a transitional state, suggesting a spreading activation of facial motor patterning. Thus, yawning may be seen as a nervous reflex loop which occurs as arousal reinforcement [31–33].

Yawning or Not: A Pathology?

Yawning occurs regularly, at a rate of about 1 or 2 per hour. When a yawn is observed during a 4D-US examination, it is obviously by chance or after very long investigation. Yawning generally appears after a period of rest, and indicates awakening. If normal swallowing is seen (much more frequent), yawning seems to offer no additional interest as an indication of harmonious brainstem maturation. Conversely, the lack of or a dysfunction in swallowing requires spending time on the collection of phasic and cyclic motor events that characterizes the ultradian fetal rhythm; thus, increasing the opportunity to notice a yawn. If the ultrasound examination suggests the absence of yawn and deglutition, it is imperative to search for mandibular hypoplasia and glossoptosis often associated with cleft palate [34].

Petrikovsky et al. [35] reported that clusters of yawning activity were observed in a series of anemic fetuses, and proposed that yawning repetitiveness helps track the fetus's anemia.

Diseases without Any Data Collected

Infants must develop safe and effective respiration and oral feeding skills soon after birth if they are to survive. For this to occur, infants must have the necessary anatomical structures and adequate central control to coordinate swallowing, ventilation, sleep and arousal. Yawning is associated with all of these behaviors [34]. Although no data have actually been collected, we have built a non-exhaustive inventory of congenital pathologies in which the research of yawning is of interest: congenital central hypoventilation syndrome (also known as Ondine's curse, after a figure from Germanic mythology) which results in hypoventilation, most pronounced during sleep, with relative insensitivity to hypercarbia and a lesser insensitivity to hypoxia, in the absence of other abnormalities of the cardiorespiratory system. Congenital central hypoventilation syndrome can be associated with Hirschsprung's disease. Abnormalities in swallowing or esophageal motility were identified in newborns with facial dysmorphism and hypotonia. This suggests a generalized abnormality of gastrointestinal motility and brainstem functioning [36, 37].

Mandibular hypoplasia is a frequently encountered craniofacial difference, and can be classified into congenital and developmental:

- Mandibulofacial dysostosis with a variety of limb abnormalities.
- Pierre Robin sequence is characterized by a posterior U-shaped cleft palate, retrognatia and glossoptosis. Several arguments favor an embryonic origin consisting of an anomaly in caudal hind brain development. Feeding disorders are the most important functional symptom. Maternal testimonies, which one of us received, seem to agree with the lack of yawning at birth and a parallel progress across the first year of life for swallowing and yawning. Also, Pierre Robin syndrome can be seen as prenatal a brainstem dysfunction responsible of the oro-facial maldevelopment that can be diagnosed at 23 weeks' gestation during a 4D-US [38, 39].
- Any syndrome (primary bilateral or unilateral growth anomalies) associated or not with temporo/mandibular joint ankylosis or aglossia/microglossia, i.e. Franceschetti syndrome, Goldenhar syndrome, Richner-Hanhart syndrome.

Moebius syndrome comprises a congenital facial diplegia and bilateral abducens nerve palsies by degenerative and involved nuclei of the VI, VII and XII nerves. Simultaneous occurrence of limb malformations with cranial nerve dysfunction suggests a disruption in normal morphogenesis during a critical period in the development of the embryonic brainstem, most likely 4–7 weeks of gestation. Instances of bilateral paresis of the soft palate and scattered instances of dysphagia (some of which resolve in infancy) have been reported. Inability to close the mouth is the norm [40, 41].

Watershed infarcts in the fetal and neonatal brainstem are clinically expressed as multiple cranial neuropathies, failure of the central respiratory drive, or dysphagia [42].

Goldenhar syndrome includes malformations primarily involving the jaw, mouth and ears and, in most cases, affects one side of the body. It represents defects in the embryonic first and second brachial arches, the first pharyngeal pouch and brachial cleft, and the primordia of the temporal bone [43].

Joubert syndrome is a rare genetic disorder characterized by the absence or underdevelopment the cerebellar vermis and a malformed brainstem. The most common features include ataxia, an abnormal breathing pattern, sleep apnea, abnormal eye and tongue movements, and hypotonia [44].

It is possible to complete this catalog by adding congenital trismus, Crisponi syndrome, Stüve-Wiedemann syndrome, and other similar disorders.

Conclusion

A popular belief states that yawning is a response to elevated CO_2 or depressed O_2 levels in the blood. Provine and Tate [45] found no support for this hypothesis. Fetal yawning in amniotic fluid (like a fish's yawn in water) also show data against any association between oxygenation capacity and yawning.

With the significant advances in the image quality and resolution of ultrasound, and now 3D and 4D technology, the practice of ultrasound examination during pregnancy has moved forward from an anatomical examination to a functional evaluation. Recognition of fetal yawning helps to verify the harmonious progress of brainstem maturation and to appreciate the neural underpinnings of the sleep and arousal systems. Abnormalities in yawning foster intensive research of anemic fetuses (frequency amplified) or brainstem dysfunction with or without mandibular hypoplasia (frequency sparse or null) [34]. We hope and expect that upcoming research completes the data currently available.

References

1 Kurjak A, Azumendi G: The Fetus in Three Dimensions: Imaging, Embryology and Fetoscopy. London, Informa Healthcare, 2007, p 520.

2 Yan F, Dai SY, Akther N, Kuno A, Yanagihara T, Hata T: Four-dimensional sonographic assessment of fetal facial expression early in the third trimester. Int J Gynaecol Obstet 2006;94:108–113.

3 Sepulveda W, Mangiamarchi M: Fetal yawning. Ultrasound Obstet Gynecol 1995;5:57–59.

4 Egerman RS, Emerson DS: Images in clinical medicine: a fetal yawn. N Engl J Med 1996;335:1497.

5 Marder E, Rehm KJ: Development of central pattern generating circuits. Curr Opin Neurobiol 2005;15: 86–93.

6 Kurjak A, Stanojevic M, Azumendi G, et al: The potential of four dimensional (4D) ultrasonography in the assessment of fetal awareness. J Perinat Med 2005;33:46–53.

7 Yigiter AB, Kavak ZN: Normal standards of fetal behavior assessed by four-dimensional sonography. J Matern Fetal Neonatal Med 2006;19:707–721.

8 de Vries JI, Visser GH, Prechtl HF: The emergence of fetal behaviour. Early Hum Dev 1982;7:301–322 and 1985;12:99–120.

9 Walusinski O, Deputte B: The phylogeny, ethology and nosogeny of yawning. Rev Neurol (Paris) 2004; 160:1011–1021.

10 Masuzaki H, Masuzaki M: Color Doppler imaging of fetal yawning. Ultrasound Obstet Gynecol 1996; 8:355–356.

11 van Woerden EE, van Geijin HP, Caron FJ, et al: Fetal mouth movements during behavioural states 1F and 2F. Eur J Obstet Gynecol Reprod Biol 1988; 29:97–105.

12 Briscoe J, Wilkinson DG: Establishing neuronal circuitry: Hox genes make the connection. Genes Dev 2004;18:1643–1648.

13 Köntges G, Lumsden A: Rhombencephalic neural crest segmentation is preserved throughout craniofacial ontogeny. Development 1996;122:3229–3242.
14 Graham A: The development and evolution of the pharyngeal arches. J Anat 2001;199:133–141.
15 Santagati F, Rijli F: Cranial neural crest and the building of the vertebrate head. Nature Rev Neurosci 2003;4:806–818.
16 Joseph R: Fetal brain behavior and cognitive development. Developmental Rev 2000;20:81–98.
17 Robinson SR, Blumberg MS, Lane MS, et al: Spontaneous motor activity in fetal and infant rats is organized into discrete multilimb bouts. Behav Neurosci 2000;114:328–336.
18 Almli CR, Ball RH, Wheeler ME: Human fetal and neonatal movements patterns: gender differences and fetal-to-neonatal continuity. Dev Psychhobiol 2001;38:252–273.
19 Jacob J, Guthrie S: Facial visceromotor neurons display specific rhombomere origin and axon pathfinding behavior. J Neurosci 2000;20:7664–7671.
20 Rose RJ: Prenatal programming of behavior: a twin-study perspective. Neurosci Biobehav Rev 2005;19: 321–327.
21 Wragg LE, Smith JA, Borden CS: Myoneural maturation and function of the fetal rat tongue at the time of secondary plate closure. Arch Oral Biol 1972;17:673–682.
22 Ezure K, Tanaka I: Convergence of central respiratory and locomotor rhythms onto single neurons of the lateral reticular nucleus. Exp Brain Res 1997; 113:230–242.
23 Siegel JM: Sleep phylogeny: clues to the evolution and function of sleep; in Luppi PH (ed): Sleep: Circuits and Functions. Boca Raton, CRC, 2005, pp 163–176.
24 Valatx JL: The ontogeny and physiology confirms the dual nature of sleep states. Arch Ital Biol 2004; 142:569–580.
25 Davis FC, Frank MG, Heller HC: Ontogeny of sleep and circadian rhythms; in Turek FW, Zee PC (eds): Regulation of Sleep and Circadian Rhythms. New York, Marcel Dekker, 1999, pp 19–79.
26 Blumberg MS, Luca DE: A developmental and component analysis of active sleep. Develop Psychobiol 1996;29:1–22.
27 Kobayashi T, Good C, Mamiya K, et al: Development of REM sleep drive and clinical implications. J Appl Physiol 2004;96:735–746.
28 Walusinski O: Yawning: from birth to senescence. Psychol Neuropsychiatr Vieil 2006;4:39–46.
29 Roodenburg PJ, Wladimiroff JW, van Es A, et al: Classification and quantitative aspects of fetal movements during the second half of normal pregnancy. Early Hum Develop 1991;25:19–35.
30 Saper CB, Chou TC, Scammell TE: The sleep switch: hypothalamic control of sleep and wakefulness. Trends Neurosci 2001;24:726–731.
31 Baenninger R: On yawning and its functions. Psychonomic Bul Rev 1997;4:198–207.
32 Giganti F, Hayes MJ, Akilesh MR, et al: Yawning and behavioral states in premature infants. Development Psychobiol 2002;41:289–293.
33 Pace-Schott EF, Hobson A: The neurobiology of sleep: genetics, cellular physiology and subcortical networks. Nature Rev Neurosci 2002;3:591–605.
34 Prechtl HFR: Qualitative changes of spontaneous movements in fetus and preterm infant are a marker of neurological dysfunction. Early Hum Dev 1990; 23:151–158.
35 Petrikovsky BM, Kaplan GP, Holsten N: Fetal yawning activity in normal and high-risk fetuses: a preliminary observation. Ultrasound Obstet Gynecol 1999;13:127–130.
36 American Thoracic Society: Idiopathic congenital central hypoventilation syndrome: diagnosis and management. Am J Respir Crit Care Med 1999;160: 368–373.
37 Kumar R, Macey PM, Woo MA, et al: Diffusion tensor imaging demonstrates brainstem and cerebellar abnormalities in congenital central hypoventilation syndrome. Pediatr Res 2008;64:275–280.
38 Abadie V, Morisseau-Durand M: Brainstem dysfunction: a possible neuroembryological pathogenesis of isolated Pierre Robin sequence. Eur J Ped 2002;161:275–280.
39 Matsumato M, Yanagihara T, Hanaoka U, Maesato T, Kuno A, Yamashiro C, Tanaka H, Hayashi K, Hata T: Antenatal three-dimensional sonographic features of Pierre-Robin syndrome: case report. Gynecol Obstet Invest 2001;51:141–142.
40 Cattaneo L, Chierici E, Bianchi B, et al: The localization of facial motor impairment in sporadic Möbius syndrome. Neurology 2006;66:1907–1912.
41 May M, Schaitkin B, Shapiro A: Facial nerve disorders in newborns and children; in May M, Schaitkin BM: The Facial Nerve, ed 2. Stuttgart, Thieme, 2000, pp 339–365.
42 Sarnat HB: Watershed infarcts in the fetal and neonatal brainstem: an aetiology of central hypoventilation, dysphagia, micrognatia. Eur J Ped Neurol 2004;8:71–87.

43 Volpe P, Gentile M: Three dimensional diagnosis of Goldenhar syndrome. Ultrasound Obstet Gyncol 2004;24:798–800.
44 Yachnis AT: Cerebellar and brainstem development: an overview in relation to Joubert syndrome. J Child Neurol 1999;14:570–573.
45 Provine RR, Tate BC, Geldmacher LL: Yawning: No effect of 3–5% CO_2. 100% O_2, and exercise. Behav Neural Biol 1987;48:382–393.

Dr. Olivier Walusinski
20 rue de Chartres
FR–28160 Brou (France)
Tel. +33 2 37 47 07 77, Fax +33 2 37 47 19 07
E-Mail walusinski@baillement.com

Walusinski O (ed): The Mystery of Yawning in Physiology and Disease.
Front Neurol Neurosci. Basel, Karger, 2010, vol 28, pp 42–46

Sleep, Sleepiness and Yawning

F. Giganti · I. Zilli · S. Aboudan · P. Salzarulo

Department of Psychology, University of Florence, Florence, Italy

Abstract

This chapter will discuss the relationship between yawning, sleep onset, awakening and sleepiness. Models concerning wake-sleep regulation will be discussed in relation to yawning. Yawning close to sleep, before and after, will be examined in several conditions and populations. Also, the time course of yawning and sleepiness assessed by subjective estimates will be described.

The relationship between spontaneous (i.e. temporally non-related to external events) yawning and sleep is obvious. Both personal experience and objective scientific evaluation support the close relationship in time between the two.

This implies that there should be some common physiological and biochemical bases. In other words, structures and substances that are implicated in the transition between waking and sleep (and vice versa) are also, at least partially, involved in yawning.

Research on yawning has yielded many possible structures and substances [1]. Clinical and pharmacological evidence indicates that the hypothalamus (mainly the paraventricular nucleus), the bulbus and the region around the pons with frontal connections are involved in triggering yawning. The numerous connections between the bulbus and the ascending reticular activating system, largely involved in the sleep-wake rhythm and the modulation of arousal levels, suggest a relationship between yawning and sleepiness.

Moreover, among the several neurotransmitters and neuropeptides that are involved in the control of yawning [2], adrenocorticotropin, α-melanocyte-stimulating hormone, acetylcholine, dopamine, nitric oxide, excitatory amino acids and oxytocin have a facilitatory effect, while serotonin and noradrenaline have different effects (facilitatory or inhibitory) according to the receptor involved; GABA and opioid peptides have an inhibitory effect. It is well known that many of these substances are involved in sleep-wake regulation.

Concerning sleep, despite long-term research that has provided information about what happens during sleep, the time course of such central nervous system activities before and after sleep is scarcely (or not at all) known; thus, limiting our understanding of the interaction between the processes regulating both yawning and its proximity to sleep.

Serotonin could be involved in the time preceding sleep onset, as we know it increases progressively before sleep [3] and decreases after motor activity stops (J. Adrien personal communication). However, for the process of awakening, much less is known.

In the 1980s, several groups showed the time course of yawning and its relationship to sleep. There is a small increase in the afternoon and a clear peak in yawning frequency in the evening before sleep onset [4]. Provine [5] showed the progressive increase in yawning frequency before sleep onset and the decrease after sleep.

It is interesting to note that the stretching that accompanies opening the mouth occurs mainly after awakening in comparison to the time preceding sleep. The 'additional' function of that component of yawning is currently unknown. Could it be a way of enhancing the vigilance level via the proprioceptive input coming from muscle contraction? This interpretation could be an argument in favor of the theory suggesting that yawning is a means of increasing arousal. This theory should be reconsidered taking into account whether the presence/absence of stretching has an impact upon the occurrence/length of sleep. Furthermore, as yawning is not always successful in counteracting sleepiness, could stretching help delay sleep? If stretching seems to occur alongside yawning after awakening to increase alertness, could it be used voluntarily to remain awake in the evening or in other circumstances? To better understand the real effect of stretching, its contribution should be evaluated in each type of person (infants, elderly, their chronotype, subjects with excessive daytime sleepiness, and so on).

The time course displayed by yawning during the day is reminiscent of models trying to explain wake-sleep regulation.

The model of Borbély [6–8], based on the effects of sleep deprivation on the time course of slow wave sleep during the sleep recovery, described the interaction of 'process S' and 'process C'. The former represents the homeostatic factor and it is linked to the progressive accumulation of the need for sleep during the waking period (sleep propensity), whereas the latter represents the circadian factor and it is linked to body temperature fluctuations. During sleep, the time course of the 'S process' is expressed by the time course of slow wave sleep, which progressively decreases during sleep.

What is the expression of the 'S process' during the waking period? Cajochen et al. [9] considered the power density in the 6.25–9.0 Hz range of the EEG collected during waking as a marker of homeostatic sleep pressure. Could yawning be considered as a behavioral expression of this sleep pressure? The higher frequency of yawning before sleep onset and particularly its progressive increase in the 3 h preceding sleep (fig. 1) suggests that yawning could be an expression of sleep pressure [10, 11]. However, in this case, how should one explain the high frequency of yawning observed upon awakening, when sleep pressure should be very low? As regards

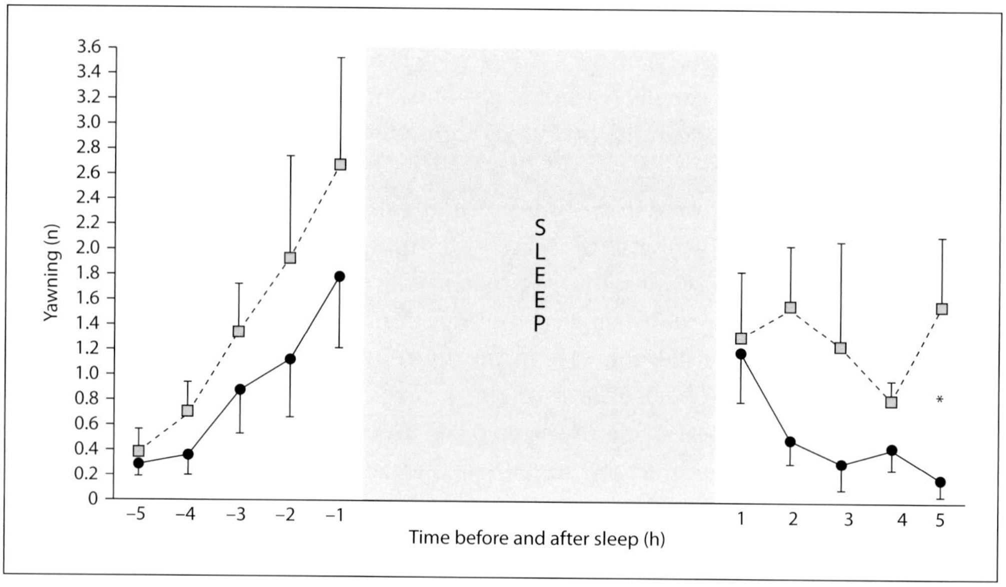

Fig. 1. Yawning frequency in evening (□) and morning (●) types before and after sleep. Data presented as means ± SE. * $p \leq 0.05$ (post hoc comparison). Reproduced with kind permission [10].

sleep regulation models, a 3-process model has been proposed, in which the wakefulness process (W) has been added to explain why subjects are usually drowsy upon awakening ('sleep inertia' effect) [12]. The sleep inertia effect could explain why the number of yawns is high upon awakening: the W process could regulate yawning in this period of the day. The influence of the circadian factor (process C) on yawning remains unclear. Experimental settings that evaluate the time course of yawning in free-running conditions (i.e. without the influences of external zeitgebers) are necessary to ascertain the circadian component of yawning occurrence.

The relationship between yawning and sleep could be approached by comparing subjects of different sleep typologies, and/or experimentally modulating some sleep characteristics.

We investigated the relation of yawning to sleep in some special populations showing unusual sleeping times or durations for their age. The time of sleeping affects yawning production [10]: evening types yawn more frequently than morning types (particularly in the morning). In morning types, the yawning frequency remains quite low during the daytime and increases in the evening, whereas in evening types it decreases throughout the day and reaches its lowest level in the early evening. However, in both types, yawning frequency progressively increases in the hours immediately preceding sleep onset, whereas after awakening evening types show a higher yawning frequency that remains quite stable in the following hours, while morning types display a decline.

The amount of sleep an individual gets does not greatly influence their yawning rate. Differences between short and long sleepers arise only after waking up in the morning, when short sleepers yawn less than long sleepers. This finding could indicate that sleep inertia dissipates more rapidly in short sleepers and their vigilance level is high quicker. Both in short and long sleepers, yawning frequency increases in the hours preceding sleep onset; nevertheless, short sleepers (notwithstanding the longer waking episode) yawn less than long sleepers. The lower frequency of yawning before sleep could indicate that those subjects have no need to resist sleeping.

The low yawning frequency after awakening highlights a difference between short sleepers and morning types: proximity to sleep is thus modulated by other subjects characteristics, like the typology.

The relationship of yawning to sleep and sleepiness has also been investigated in the elderly [11]. Older subjects yawn less than young ones, mainly in the morning and in the mid-afternoon.

Old people, like young people, yawn mainly after awakening and before sleep, but show an earlier morning peak and evening rise. In all adults, the time course of yawning parallels the time course of sleepiness, except upon awakening when the number of yawns does not correspond to a high level of sleepiness. These results suggest that sleepiness and the proximity to sleep could independently influence yawning production.

In conclusion, the relationship between yawning, sleep and sleepiness seems evident both from physiological and behavioral perspectives. The relationship between yawning, proximity to sleep, and sleepiness is steady before sleep onset, but not after sleep. However, the increase in yawning frequency before sleep onset has been found in two sleep typologies and in the elderly; the frequency and time course of yawning upon awakening are different as a function of sleep typology and age.

Further experimental studies are necessary. For example, it could be useful to evaluate yawning frequency and time after experimentally induced changes to the time and amount of sleeping (partial sleep restriction or total deprivation), and to use a fine-grained analysis of the time course of both yawning occurrence and sleepiness to ascertain if yawning can be considered a behavioral expression of sleep pressure.

References

1 Aubin HJ, Garma L: Le Bâillement. Psychiatry Psychobiol 1988;3:275–286.
2 Argiolas A, Melis MR: The neuropharmacology of yawning. Eur J Pharmacol 1998;343:1–16.
3 Jouvet M: Sérotonine et sommeil, une histoire inachevée. Med Sci 1995;11:886–893.
4 Baenninger R, Binkley S, Baenninger M: Field observations of yawning and activity in humans. Physiol Behav 1996;59:421–425.
5 Provine RR: Yawning. Am Sci 2005;93:532–539.
6 Borbély A: A two process model of sleep regulation. Hum Neurobiol 1982;1:195–204.
7 Daan S, Beersma DG, Borbély AA: Timing of human sleep: recovery process gated by a circadian pacemaker. Am J Physiol 1984;246:161–183.
8 Achermann P, Borbély AA: Simulation of human sleep: ultradian dynamics of electroencephalographic slow-wave activity. J Biol Rhythms 1990;5: 141–157.

9 Cajochen C, Brunner D, Krauchi K, Graw P, Wirz Justice A: Power density in theta alpha frequency of the waking EEG progressively increases during sustained wakefulness. Sleep 1995;18:890–894.

10 Zilli I, Giganti F, Salzarulo P: Yawning in morning and evening types. Physiol Behav 2007;91:218–222.

11 Zilli I, Giganti F, Uga V: Yawning and subjective sleepiness in the elderly. J Sleep Res 2008;17:303–308.

12 Åkerstedt T, Folkard S: The three process model of alertness and its extension to performance, sleep latency and sleep length. Chronobiol 1997;14:115–123.

Fiorenza Giganti
Department of Psychology, University of Florence
Via di San Salvi 12, Complesso di San Salvi, Padiglione 26
IT–50135 Florence (Italy)
Tel. +39 055 6237853, Fax +39 055 6236047, E-Mail fiorenza.giganti@unifi.it

Walusinski O (ed): The Mystery of Yawning in Physiology and Disease.
Front Neurol Neurosci. Basel, Karger, 2010, vol 28, pp 47–54

Interplay between Yawning and Vigilance: A Review of the Experimental Evidence

Adrian G. Guggisberg[a] · Johannes Mathis[b] · Christian W. Hess[b]

[a]Department of Clinical Neurosciences, University of Geneva, Geneva, and [b]Department of Neurology, Inselspital, University of Bern, Bern, Switzerland

Abstract

Background: Yawning is a phylogenetically old behavior of ubiquitous occurrence. The origin and function of this conspicuous phenomenon have been subject to speculation for centuries. A widely held hypothesis posits that yawning increases the arousal level during sleepiness; thus, providing a homeostatic regulation of vigilance. **Methods:** This chapter reviews experimental data on the relationship between yawning and vigilance that allow testing of the components and predictions of this hypothesis. **Results:** Behavioral studies and electroencephalographic (EEG) recordings of brain activity before and after yawning have provided consistent evidence that yawning occurs during states of low vigilance; thus, substantiating the notion that it is provoked by sleepiness. However, studies analyzing autonomic nervous activity and EEG-based indices of vigilance in yawning subjects did not find specific autonomic activations or increased arousal levels after yawning. **Conclusions:** The data therefore do not support an arousing effect of yawning or a role in regulation of vigilance or autonomic tone.

Yawning is a conspicuous behavior that can be observed in numerous animal species from fetal stages to old age. It is therefore not surprising that the question of what might be its cause and function has always aroused human curiosity.

For several centuries, at least since Hippocrates in the 4th century BC, scholars have attributed a respiratory function to yawning: it was thought that it increases oxygen levels in the brain [1, 2]. However, yawning would be a much less effective way of increasing oxygen intake than rapid breathing, especially since the deep inspiration during yawning is followed by a period of relative apnea [3]. Indeed, experiments by Provine et al. [4] have demonstrated that healthy subjects who are exposed to gas mixtures with high levels of CO_2 increase their breathing rate, but do not yawn more frequently.

Nevertheless, the idea that yawning might play an important role in regulating individual brain physiology has remained in the literature even after the rejection of the respiratory hypotheses. A widely expressed proposition has speculated that yawning might be responsible for the homeostatic regulation of vigilance and brain arousal level [3, 5].

In this chapter, we review studies and experiments that have empirically assessed the functional relationship between yawning and vigilance. A mechanism that is capable of regulating brain activation would need at least 2 different components: an afferent loop that responds to states of low vigilance, and an efferent loop that acts on the brain arousal level. Accordingly, the vigilance hypothesis makes 2 different predictions that can be empirically tested: (1) yawning is triggered by drowsiness, and (2) yawning arouses the brain.

Before examining experimental data on these predictions, we will summarize different methods that allow the measurement of vigilance and arousal associated with yawning.

Measuring Vigilance

Arousal is a global activation of brain activity that progresses from brain stem structures to centers of the autonomic nervous system and to distributed cortical areas [6, 7]. The resulting autonomic and cortical activations can be assessed with non-invasive techniques.

The gold standard for non-invasive measurement of cortical activity is electroencephalography (EEG). Spontaneous brain activity produces electromagnetic oscillations in a variety of frequencies, which in turn correlate with specific aspects of human vigilance and arousal. Delta frequencies (<3 Hz) are known to increase with the duration of wakefulness and to decrease during sleep, and are therefore interpreted as an indicator of an individual's sleep pressure [8]. In addition, low-frequency activity below ~6 Hz increases in anterior and central brain areas during the transition from wakefulness to sleep, and reaches a maximum over the fronto-central midline during drowsiness [9–11]. Alpha oscillations (approx. 8–12 Hz) have maximal amplitude when the recorded subject is awake, at rest, and has the eyes closed. Sleepiness is associated with a decrease and slowing of alpha activity, and with a topographical shift in an anterior direction along the midline of the scalp [9, 10, 12]. Increased arousal levels are also manifested by an attenuation of alpha oscillations in EEG, but, in contrast to sleepiness, they also induce an acceleration of alpha frequencies [13, 14].

Fluctuations in autonomous nervous activity produce, among other things, changes in heart rate [15] and sympathetic nerve activity [16], both of which were measured in studies of yawning.

Skin conductance was also shown to be a reliable indicator of the arousal level, reflecting both autonomic and cortical activities [13, 17].

Experimental Yawn Induction

Behavioral as well as electrophysiological analyses require a sufficient quantity of observable yawns. Several techniques have therefore been applied to induce yawning in test subjects.

In humans, yawning has a pronounced contagious effect which is frequently used for experimental purposes. Videos or photographs of yawning persons are shown to study participants who are recruited for analysis of yawning.

Yawning also occurs more frequently during boredom, and boring texts have been found to facilitate yawns [18].

Several studies interested in the relationship between yawning and vigilance have used sleepy subjects for their analyses [19–21], since the arousal hypothesis predicts that they yawn particularly often.

A vigilance test commonly used in clinical practice to evaluate the ability of patients to stay awake proved to be a useful tool for the investigation of yawning. The Maintenance of Wakefulness Test is a standardized test during which the subjects must try to stay awake while sitting alone in a quiet and darkened room [22, 23]. The test thus combines sleepiness with boredom and frequently induces yawning.

Yawning Occurs Preferentially during Drowsiness

Behavioral and neurophysiological studies provide converging evidence that yawning occurs preferentially during periods of drowsiness.

The frequency of yawning has a distinctive circadian distribution and occurs most frequently before and after sleep [24, 25], i.e. during periods of lower levels of vigilance and alertness. Furthermore, the yawning rate correlates with the individual's subjective feeling of drowsiness [28] and adjusts to individual circadian rhythms [26–28]. See also contribution by Giganti et al. (this volume, pp. 42–46) for further details on this aspect.

If yawning is triggered by drowsiness, we should be able to observe corresponding physiological signs of sleepiness before yawns. We used electroencephalography (EEG) to test this in human subjects. Indeed, delta power density over central midline brain areas (which is thought to represent sleep pressure and sleepiness) was found to be significantly greater before yawns than before control movements without yawning [19]. Thus, sleep pressure and drowsiness were significantly greater when subjects yawned than when they only moved. This finding provides further evidence for the notion that yawns are triggered by drowsiness.

Yawning Does Not Produce Arousal

The arousal hypothesis predicts that yawning reduces sleepiness or increases the arousal level. Several studies have tested this prediction by investigating spectral EEG changes and markers of autonomic activity after yawns in humans. However, no corresponding evidence could be found.

Laing and Ogilvie [20] recorded the EEG of healthy human subjects who spontaneously yawned before going to sleep. Thirty-second samples of EEG before and after yawns from 4 participants were subjected to a spectral analysis. Spectral power in the theta, alpha, or spindle frequency bands did not significantly change after yawning. Furthermore, EEG power in these bands before and after yawning was not significantly different from EEG power before and after postural adjustments without yawning.

In a second study by this research group, analyses were extended to a larger population of 12 subjects and to more frequency bands. Again, no lasting changes in EEG activity attributable to yawning could be observed when pre- and post-yawn samples were compared. Transient decreases in delta activity as well as transient increases in theta, spindle, and beta activity were noted, but they only reached significance when the analysis was a priori limited to data segments between 10 and 20 s before and after yawning [21].

We analyzed EEG recordings of 16 patients who underwent Maintenance of Wakefulness Tests to elucidate the origin of excessive daytime sleepiness or non-restorative sleep and who had yawned at least 4 times during the test [19]. None of the included subjects had brain lesions, metabolic disorders or hormonal disorders that could have affected the physiological mechanisms underlying yawning. We observed that the increase in delta power over the vertex that was observed before yawning (as compared to delta activity before postural adjustments without yawning) persisted to the same amount after yawning. Thus, yawning did not reverse the increased sleep pressure and drowsiness that seemed to have triggered it. The EEG after yawning even showed a pattern that is typical of a decreased [9, 10, 12] rather an increased arousal level: alpha rhythms decreased, decelerated and shifted towards central brain regions after yawning, as compared to the data segments before yawning. Conversely, we did observe EEG markers of increased arousal levels after simple postural adjustments. Alpha rhythms became faster and smaller after body movements, a pattern that is qualitatively similar as – but quantitatively smaller than – the spectral changes that can be observed 30 min after oral ingestion of 250 mg caffeine [13]. Hence, if yawning had had an arousing effect – even if it were as small as the effect of simple postural adjustments – we would have detected it with our EEG analyses. Instead, we observed signs of progressive drowsiness after yawning.

Several studies have observed that yawning is followed by increases in heart rate, i.e. by activation of the autonomic system. However, this activation occurs to the same amount after simple movements without yawning or during respiration. It is therefore entirely unspecific and related to the associated movement and respiration rather than yawning as such [15, 19]. In other words, the act of yawning does not induce more autonomic changes than the ones that already occur hundreds of times throughout the day due to simple breathing or moving. Hence, from an evolutionary perspective, yawning does not provide an advantage with regards to autonomic activity, and it therefore does not make sense to attribute an autonomic function to yawning.

Other studies have assessed the arousal level after yawning by measuring the skin conductance [13, 17]. Again, no specific increase in skin conductance was found after yawning in one study [15], and another study even observed a yawning-induced decrease in skin conductance, i.e. a decrease in arousal level [29].

Arousal reactions associated with yawning have been observed in anesthetized rats [30–32], but this arousal started before, not after, the actual yawning. It can therefore not be interpreted as a consequence of yawning, but rather corresponds to a requirement for yawning to occur during anesthesia. Indeed, yawning almost never spontaneously occurs during sleep [24–26]. Another study has inferred yawning-related arousals from recordings of the bispectral index in humans during induction of anesthesia [33]. However, the bispectral index is sensitive to contaminations from cranial muscle activity which is abundant during yawning. Even if the observations of the study did not result from contaminations, the same interpretation holds as for the data obtained in rats.

One of the arguments for an arousing effect of yawning has been the observation that yawns are associated with a significant increase in motor activity [3, 34]. However, motor activity depends on numerous factors and does not necessarily correlate with the cerebral arousal level. Based on our observation of an arousing effect of body movements, we have suggested that the increased motor activity observed after yawning may not be an indicator of an arousing effect of yawning, but an effective countermeasure against the underlying drowsiness [19].

Discussion

The experimental data suggest that yawning indeed occurs during progressive drowsiness, which is compatible with the notion that it is triggered by states of low vigilance. However, numerous studies using various experimental techniques were unable to observe a specific arousing effect of yawning on the brain or the autonomic nervous system.

It might be argued that the arousing effect of yawning was not accessible to EEG recordings or measurements of autonomic activity. However, vigilance changes are typically manifested diffusely over the whole brain, and EEG is considered the gold standard to measure it. Moreover, even small arousing reactions, such as the ones induced by simple body movements, could be detected.

Another argument might postulate that the arousing effect of yawning occurred with a delay that was greater than the 10- to 30-second post-yawn period analyzed in the different studies. However, central regulation mechanisms typically respond with a much shorter latency than 30 s, and it would be unclear why in the case of vigilance regulation it would 'wait' for such a long time. Furthermore, the non-significant changes of the EEG during the first seconds after yawning points to decreased rather than increased arousal levels.

In contrast to the lack of direct empirical evidence for an arousing effect of yawning, an increasing number of studies have accumulated evidence for an important social function, at least in humans. Yawning has a strong contagious effect in humans and primates. The susceptibility to contagious yawning correlates with social skills in healthy subjects [35] and is reduced in patients with disorders affecting the ability of social interaction, such as autism [36] and schizophrenia [37]. Furthermore, watching other persons yawn activates brain regions related to empathy and social behavior [38–41]. These findings suggest that the regulating function of yawning might not take place in individuals but rather be effective in social groups. Thus, yawning may be a non-verbal form of communication that helps synchronize the behavior within groups [42–45].

Despite some progress in yawning research in the last few years, yawning remains insufficiently understood to establish a generally accepted model of the origin and purpose of yawning. More data on the neural and pharmacological processes that precede, accompany and follow yawns are needed. Given the relatively solid evidence for social yawns, future research should also address the anatomical connections and functional interactions between social cortical networks and centers responsible for yawning control.

Acknowledgments

The authors would like to thank Olivier Walusinski for his invaluable online archive of articles on yawning which greatly facilitated the literature research for this chapter.

References

1 Trautmann R: Le bâillement. Bordeaux, Thesis, 1901.
2 Schiller F: Yawning? J Hist Neurosci 2002;11:392–401.
3 Baenninger R: On yawning and its functions. Psychonomic Bul Rev 1997;4:198–207.
4 Provine RR, Tate BC, Geldmacher LL: Yawning: no effect of 3–5% CO_2, 100% O_2, and exercise. Behav Neural Biol 1987;48:382–393.
5 Walusinski O, Deputte BL: Le bâillement : phylogenèse, éthologie, nosogénie. Rev Neurol (Paris) 2004; 160:1011–1021.
6 Moruzzi G, Magoun HW: Brain stem reticular formation and activation of the EEG. Electroencephalogr Clin Neurophysiol 1949;1:455–473.
7 Sforza E, Jouny C, Ibanez V: Cardiac activation during arousal in humans: further evidence for hierarchy in the arousal response. Clin Neurophysiol 2000;111:1611–1619.
8 Borbely AA, Baumann F, Brandeis D, Strauch I, Lehmann D: Sleep deprivation: effect on sleep stages and EEG power density in man. Electroencephalogr Clin Neurophysiol 1981;51:483–495.

9 De Gennaro L, Ferrara M, Bertini M: The boundary between wakefulness and sleep: quantitative electroencephalographic changes during the sleep onset period. Neuroscience 2001;107:1–11.
10 De Gennaro L, Ferrara M, Curcio G, Cristiani R: Antero-posterior EEG changes during the wakefulness-sleep transition. Clin Neurophysiol 2001;112: 1901–1911.
11 Tanaka H, Hayashi M, Hori T: Topographical characteristics of slow wave activities during the transition from wakefulness to sleep. Clin Neurophysiol 2000;111:417–427.
12 Tanaka H, Hayashi M, Hori T: Topographical characteristics and principal component structure of the hypnagogic EEG. Sleep 1997;20:523–534.
13 Barry RJ, Rushby JA, Wallace MJ, Clarke AR, Johnstone SJ, Zlojutro I: Caffeine effects on resting-state arousal. Clin Neurophysiol 2005;116:2693–2700.
14 Barry RJ, Clarke AR, McCarthy R, Selikowitz M, Rushby JA, Ploskova E: EEG differences in children as a function of resting-state arousal level. Clin Neurophysiol 2004;115:402–408.
15 Greco M, Baenninger R: Effects of yawning and related activities on skin conductance and heart rate. Physiol Behav 1991;50:1067–1069.
16 Askenasy JJ, Askenasy N: Inhibition of muscle sympathetic nerve activity during yawning. Clin Auton Res 1996;6:237–239.
17 Lawrence CA, Barry RJ, Clarke AR, Johnstone SJ, McCarthy R, Selikowitz M, Broyd SJ: Methylphenidate effects in attention deficit/hyperactivity disorder: electrodermal and ERP measures during a continuous performance task. Psychopharmacology (Berl) 2005;183:81–91.
18 Provine RR, Hamernik HB: Yawning: effects of stimulus interest. Bull Psychon Soc 1986;24:437–438.
19 Guggisberg AG, Mathis J, Herrmann US, Hess CW: The functional relationship between yawning and vigilance. Behav Brain Res 2007;179:159–166.
20 Laing JV, Ogilvie RD: EEG correlates of yawning during sleep onset. Sleep Res 1988;17:98.
21 Regehr KL, Ogilvie RD, Simons IA: Electrophysiological correlates of yawning. Sleep Res 1992; 21:14.
22 Doghramji K, Mitler MM, Sangal RB, Shapiro C, Taylor S, Walsleben J, Belisle C, Erman MK, Hayduk R, Hosn R, O'Malley EB, Sangal JM, Schutte SL, Youakim JM: A normative study of the maintenance of wakefulness test (MWT). Electroencephalogr Clin Neurophysiol 1997;103:554–562.
23 Littner MR, Kushida C, Wise M, Davila DG, Morgenthaler T, Lee-Chiong T, Hirshkowitz M, Daniel LL, Bailey D, Berry RB, Kapen S, Kramer M: Practice parameters for clinical use of the multiple sleep latency test and the maintenance of wakefulness test. Sleep 2005;28:113–121.
24 Greco M, Baenninger R, Govern J: On the context of yawning: when, where, and why? Psychol Rec 1993;43:175–183.
25 Provine RR, Hamernik HB, Curchack BC: Yawning: relation to sleeping and stretching in humans. Ethology 1987;76:152–160.
26 Giganti F, Hayes MJ, Cioni G, Salzarulo P: Yawning frequency and distribution in preterm and near term infants assessed throughout 24-h recordings. Infant Behav Dev 2007;30:641–647.
27 Zilli I, Giganti F, Salzarulo P: Yawning in morning and evening types. Physiol Behav 2007;91:218–222.
28 Zilli I, Giganti F, Uga V: Yawning and subjective sleepiness in the elderly. J Sleep Res 2008;17:303–308.
29 Baenninger R, Greco M: Some antecedents and consequences of yawning. Psychol Rec 1991;41:453–460.
30 Sato-Suzuki I, Kita I, Oguri M, Arita H: Stereotyped yawning responses induced by electrical and chemical stimulation of paraventricular nucleus of the rat. J Neurophysiol 1998;80:2765–2775.
31 Kita I, Sato-Suzuki I, Oguri M, Arita H: Yawning responses induced by local hypoxia in the paraventricular nucleus of the rat. Behav Brain Res 2000;117: 119–126.
32 Seki Y, Sato-Suzuki I, Kita I, Oguri M, Arita H: Yawning/cortical activation induced by microinjection of histamine into the paraventricular nucleus of the rat. Behav Brain Res 2002;134:75–82.
33 Kasuya Y, Murakami T, Oshima T, Dohi S: Does yawning represent a transient arousal-shift during intravenous induction of general anesthesia? Anesth Analg 2005;101:382–384.
34 Giganti F, Hayes MJ, Akilesh MR, Salzarulo P: Yawning and behavioral states in premature infants. Dev Psychobiol 2002;41:289–296.
35 Platek SM, Critton SR, Myers TE, Gallup GG: Contagious yawning: the role of self-awareness and mental state attribution. Brain Res Cogn Brain Res 2003;17:223–227.
36 Senju A, Maeda M, Kikuchi Y, Hasegawa T, Tojo Y, Osanai H: Absence of contagious yawning in children with autism spectrum disorder. Biol Lett 2007; 3:706–708.
37 Haker H, Rossler W: Empathy in schizophrenia: impaired resonance. Eur Arch Psychiatry Clin Neurosci 2009;259:352–361.

38 Platek SM, Mohamed FB, Gallup GG Jr.: Contagious yawning and the brain. Brain Res Cogn Brain Res 2005;23:448–452.
39 Schurmann M, Hesse MD, Stephan KE, Saarela M, Zilles K, Hari R, Fink GR: Yearning to yawn: the neural basis of contagious yawning. Neuroimage 2005;24:1260–1264.
40 Nahab FB, Hattori N, Saad ZS, Hallett M: Contagious yawning and the frontal lobe: an fMRI study. Hum Brain Mapp 2009;30:1744–1751.
41 Arnott SR, Singhal A, Goodale MA: An investigation of auditory contagious yawning. Cogn Affect Behav Neurosci 2009;9:335–342.
42 Barbizet J: Yawning. J Neurol Neurosurg Psychiatry 1958;21:203–209.
43 Provine RR: Yawning as a stereotyped action pattern and releasing stimulus. Ethology 1986;72:109–122.
44 Weller MP: Yawning. Lancet 1988;1:950.
45 Deputte BL: Ethological study of yawning in primates. 1. Quantitative analysis and study of causation in two species of old world monkeys (*Cercocebus albigena* and *Macaca fascicularis*). Ethology 1994;98:221–245.

Adrian G. Guggisberg
Department of Clinical Neurosciences, University of Geneva
Avenue de Beau-Séjour 26
CH–1211 Geneva 14 (Switzerland)
Tel. +41 22 382 35 21, Fax +41 22 382 36 44, E-Mail aguggis@gmail.com

Walusinski O (ed): The Mystery of Yawning in Physiology and Disease.
Front Neurol Neurosci. Basel, Karger, 2010, vol 28, pp 55–62

The Hidden Sexuality of the Yawn and the Future of Chasmology

Wolter Seuntjens

Brussels, Belgium

Abstract

Chasmology is the scientific study of yawning. Though its official history started only recently, its unofficial history stretches back to antiquity. This chapter outlines the history and current state of chasmology, through textual research and analysis, and offers a vision of its future. Particular emphasis is placed upon the author's favorite theory: the hidden sexuality of the human yawn. The 'First Law of Chasmology' states that a yawn occurs: (1) if the yawner cannot do what he would like to do, or (2) if the yawner must do something that he would rather not do. The 'Second Law of Chasmology', which is a special instance of the more general First Law, states that the yawn has an erotic and even a sexual aspect. A critical mass of proof for the validity of this Second Law is derived from various sciences and disciplines, ranging from theology and (the history of) art to ethology and pharmacology. The process of evidencing the Second Law has also established chasmology as an emerging science, i.e. a science that uses the data and information of primary sciences to make a synthesis that transforms and transcends the original scope and results of the auxiliary disciplines. The Second Law allows at least two concrete predictions about future corroborations or refutations in chasmological research. **Conclusion:** Chasmology has a bright future and may yield some surprising results in the near future.

> I don't need to believe much about yawning in order to desire to yawn
> *Richard Swinburne* [1]

Although the yawn has always aroused curiosity, it is only recently that yawning has been studied in a scientific way. Since the 1980s, more systematic research – especially physiological, psychological, ethological and pharmacological research – has cast light on the yawn. Even more recently, these combined efforts to study yawning have been given a name: chasmology. Though the name is new there were, of course, chasmologists avant la lettre. Hippocrates and Aristotle, Sennert and Boerhaave, Charcot and Trautmann and many others can be enlisted as honorary chasmologists. In this short chapter, I will only be able to outline the past, present and future of chasmology, and in doing this I will place special emphasis on the theory that I proposed in my dissertation [2].

Historical Trends and Currents

In the history of thinking about the yawn, one may discern certain fundamental approaches. I will summarily discuss these approaches concentrating on only three: the animistic, the psychological and the physiological.

Animistic

It is clear that the yawn was, and sometimes still is, regarded in an animistic vein: the yawn enables a demon to enter the body of the yawner or permits the soul to escape that same body. The animistic current probably spawned the near-universal taboo on yawning. This is the reason why people perform so many and such varied actions to avert the dangers of yawning, for example making the sign of the cross over the mouth. However, it is also possible that the animistic idea itself is an offshoot of another, an even more fundamental taboo. A subcategory of the animistic idea is expressed in the words of Emile Cioran [3]: 'According to a Christian legend, the world was born when the Devil yawned.'

It would be interesting to see if theologians could make a contribution to chasmology, taking Cioran's remark as their starting point. Another possible question to solve by theologians is whether prelapsarian man did indeed yawn (fig. 1). For as Saint Augustine said [4]: '[…] It was, in fact, after the sin that this lust arose.'

Physiological

Nowadays, many people associate yawning with a lack of oxygen. Generally, this deficiency is supposed to be in the brain. The oxygen-deficiency theory also comes in another version: an overabundance of carbon dioxide. Both the so-called hypoxia and hypercapnia theories remained unchallenged and were considered to be common sense for a long time. When these popular theories were finally tested by Provine et al. [5] in the 1980s, they were roundly refuted. A current physiological theory proposes that yawning may be a thermoregulatory mechanism providing compensatory cooling [6]. It remains to be seen whether this rather broad and bold hypothesis will stand up to critical scrutiny.

Psychological

At the psychological level, the yawn has been associated with boredom at least since Roman times. Boredom, however, is a very complex idea. Nevertheless, even if it is only partially connected with yawning, boredom may still be an interesting concept for chasmology. However, something more than boredom must be invoked to explain the following yawning bout: Hans Schnier is meeting his father for the first time in 3 years and for the first time ever they are having a serious conversation together; then Hans starts yawning [7]:

> I suddenly had to yawn. It was rude, but I couldn't help it, and I was fully aware of the discourtesy. […] I was all worked up, but dead tired, and I was sorry I had to yawn at that particular moment. […] My yawning became almost a cramp, my jaw muscles cracked.

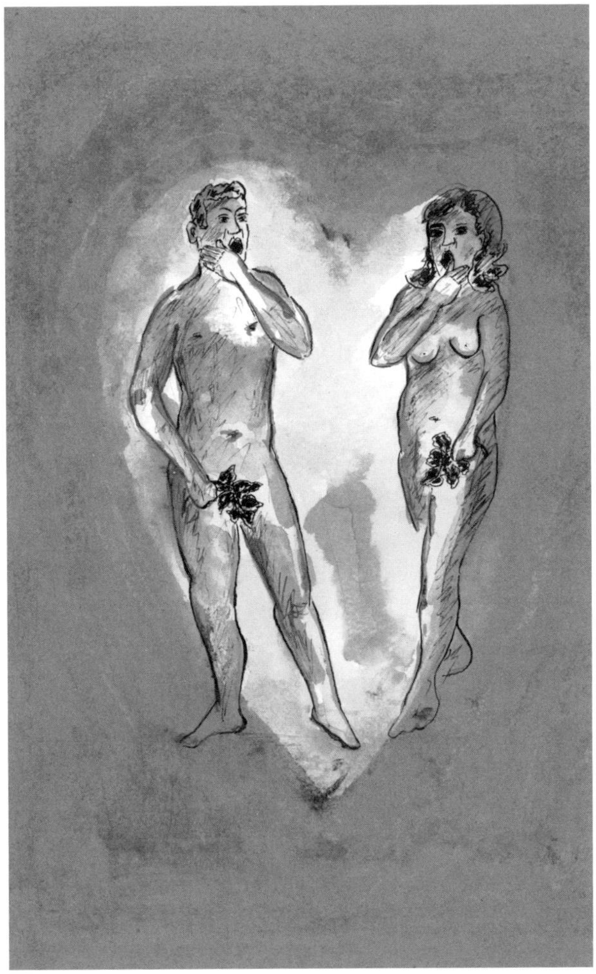

Fig. 1. Reiner Schlecker: *Yawning Adam, Yawning Eve*. 2004 (reproduced with kind permission from Reiner Schlecker).

The narrator himself – and probably the author, Heinrich Böll, too – was surprised by this inappropriate and incessant yawning in front of his father. To explain such surprising behavior, I called upon the situational description that the German physician Valentin Dumpert gave en passant in his 1921 article [8], which is best conveyed in the form of a thought experiment. Picture yourself late at night entertaining guests. Now you want to go to sleep. When there is a 'boring' guest who does not go home or if your companions do not let you go to bed, then you will yawn. However, as soon as the guest has left and you can go to sleep, the moment you can take off your clothes you will cease to yawn. Once you are in bed, it is quite unlikely that you will yawn again. In the morning we can observe, introspectively or in another person present, the same phenomenon: as long as you are happy to stay in bed you will not yawn. However, if you, rather unwillingly, must get up in order to start the day you may yawn. You will do this even when you are still lying motionless in your bed. This thought experiment poses a problem for a purely physiological explanation of the yawn. Therefore, we need a more general principle. In my book, I called this the First Law of Chasmology: a yawn will occur: (1) if the yawner cannot do what he would like to do, or (2) if the yawner must do something that he would rather not do [9].

Chasmology as an Emergent Science

Another rather ambitious approach to chasmology is to see what the primary sciences can tell us about yawning and then use this information for a seminal synthesis. The primary sciences thus become auxiliary disciplines. This ideal of chasmology is therefore to become an emergent science that transforms and transcends the basic scope and results of the auxiliary disciplines.

The Second Law of Chasmology – a special adaptation of the general First Law and a subcategory of this more ambitious approach – states that the disparate data derived from the primary sciences allow the hypothesis of the erotic/sexual aspect of the yawn.

Let us review briefly the findings of the primary sciences that allow the conjecture of what the Abbé de Lignac called intuitively 'the tedious sensuality of the yawn' [10].

Linguistic

I found that both the 'yawn' and the 'stretch' of the stretch-yawn syndrome (SYS) are semantically and etymologically associated with 'desire' and 'longing for'. A fine example is presented by the troubadours of 12th century France who used the yawn as a sign of love [11]: 'Love makes him stretch his arms, and yawn this softly.'

The association of yawning, stretching and (being in) love is also echoed by modern writers like W.B. Yeats and Ezra Pound [12].

Social-Ethnological

In several proverbs and sayings, yawning – especially contagious yawning – is interpreted as a sign of sympathy, and even of being in love. Also, in folktales the association between contagious yawning and the erotic is made [13].

Psychological

Its contagiousness is probably the most striking feature of the yawn, and over time yawning has been found to be contagious in more and more species [14, 15]. Moreover, not only is yawning contagious within, but also between species [16]. Contagious yawning is associated with empathy [17], and more specifically with sympathy. In short, the infected yawner has a positive relation with or attitude towards the original yawner.

Ethological

Yawning appears to have a much greater role in animal communication than previously thought. As sex and procreation play such important parts in animal life, it will come as no surprise that yawning can be linked with, e.g. arousal, ejaculation, orgasm (sexual response; SR). The role of yawning and especially contagious yawning in primates is receiving greater attention. However, the yawn may also be associated with the erotic or even the sexual in other orders and other classes. For instance, in birds [18]:

> The male raven's yawn puts rival males to flight or exasperates them, but attracts female ravens. Ceremonial yawning plays a big part in the love-play of cormorants and gannets, showing the yellow or black colour (respectively) for a longer or shorter time.

In dogs, when they are forced to practise repetitive and monotonous training exercises, yawning can be associated with penile erection [19].

Karl Kraus remarked: 'When animals yawn they have a human face' [20]. Is this funny because we think the opposite statement is true: 'When humans yawn they look like animals?' or are they – double paradox – both true?

Pathological

Yawning is associated with SR in a number of pathological states. In epilepsy, both yawning and SR can be part of the aura [21–23]. Spontaneous ejaculation and yawning in the final stages of rabies have been reported [24, 25].

Pharmacological

There have been many reports about paradoxical sexual side effects of psychopharmaca and especially of antidepressant drugs [26]. It has been suggested that about 5% of patients experience these. In a few cases, yawning and SR were explicitly linked. The most dramatic case concerned the causal link of yawning and orgasm in a woman who used clomipramine [27]. Every time the woman yawned – even if voluntarily – she experienced orgasm. In the heroine withdrawal syndrome ('cold turkey'), yawning and spontaneous SR are also reported [28]. Several molecules, of which oxytocin and nitric oxide are the most prominent, seem to be involved in both yawning and SR.

Arts

In many cases, artists seem to be better observers than scientists. However, the artist himself is often unaware of the significance of his observation.

In literature, we encounter many intimations of erotic yawning. Two examples will suffice to convey the general idea. The Hungarian writer Dezső Kosztolányi suggested a clear association between the yawn and the erotic [29]:

> A chambermaid yawned with the divine promise of casual love.

And Dutch novelist Margriet de Moor wrote equally convincingly [30]:

> Again our shoes lay strewn across the floor. We drank from the same glass. Gasparo stretched, yawning, and I knew what this signified: I'm getting in the mood. That afternoon everything was just right.

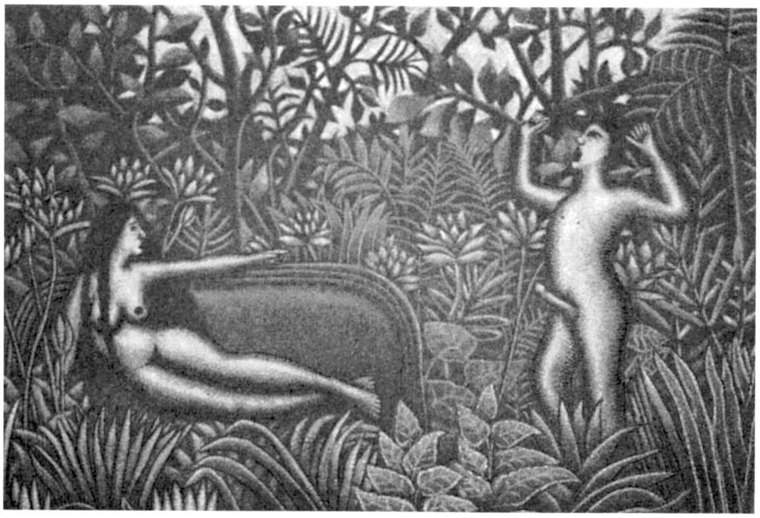

Fig. 2. Trevor Price, *Morning Yawning,* 2001 (reproduced with kind permission from Trevor Price).

In the visual arts, we encounter a phenomenon that I coined 'posture X', which opens new vistas on the yawn [2]. In (semi-)posture X (one or) two hands are raised or held behind the neck or the head. Posture X mimics the SYS. It is the substitute of the socially unacceptable SYS. Posture X is therefore the abbreviation of the technically difficult, the esthetically disturbing and, moreover, the tabooed yawn. Or, to use one more analogy concerning this 'fortunate junction of the visible and the audible', as the sigh is the auditory proxy of the yawn, so is posture X its visual proxy:

posture X → stretch → SYS → yawn

In short, posture X refers – via the stretch and the SYS – to the yawn. Thus, we find ourselves in the fortunate position of being able to study the relatively scarce yawn indirectly via the omnipresent posture X. Examples of (semi-)posture X range from the *Sleeping Ariadne of the Vatican* over Michelangelo's *Dying Captive* and Goya's *La Maja* to Matisse's *Blue Nude* and innumerable reclining, sitting and standing Venusses, putti, dancers, etc. (fig. 2).

Predictions

The theory of the erotic/sexual aspect of yawning may be corroborated or refuted in at least two ways. Firstly, it may be possible through ever more advanced scanning techniques to establish that the brain structures that are involved in SR are also involved in SYS. Secondly, it may be possible to find or make a substance that has the paradoxical sexual side effect of some drugs as its main effect: yawning causes SR.

Conclusions

As a first conclusion, we may state that chasmology has shown that yawning is not a trivial and insignificant behavior. On the contrary, yawning is a behavior pregnant with meaning. Moreover, Reber's law applies perfectly: the closer the yawn is examined, the more complex it is seen to be [31]. A second conclusion may be that there is sufficient evidence to conclude that yawning has an erotic/sexual aspect. Finally, we may assume that chasmology as an orthodox interdisciplinary science has a bright future and that as an emergent science it may yield some highly surprising results.

> 'I have not read them', said Neigh, secretly wrestling with his jaw,
> to prevent a yawn; 'but I suppose I must.'
> *Thomas Hardy [32]*

References

1 Swinburne R: The Evolution of the Soul (1986). Oxford, Oxford University Press, 1997, p 264.

2 Seuntjens W: On Yawning or The Hidden Sexuality of the Human Yawn; PhD Dissertation, Vrije Universiteit, Amsterdam, 2004, Brou/Veghel, Editions Oscitatio, 2004.

3 Cioran EM: Tears and Saints (1937). Chicago, University of Chicago, 1995, p 53.

4 St. Augustine: The City of God (tr. Henry Bettenson: book XIV, chapter 21). London, Penguin, 2003, p 583.

5 Provine RR, Tate BC, Geldmacher LL: Yawning: no effect of 3–5% CO_2, 100% O_2, and exercise. Behav Neural Biol 1987;48:382–393.

6 Gallup AC, Gallup GG: Yawning and thermoregulation. Physiol Behav 2008;95:10–16.

7 Böll H: The Clown (1967). Harmondsworth, Penguin, 1994, p 144.

8 Dumpert V: Zur Kenntnis des Wesens und der physiologischen Bedeutung des Gähnens. J Psychol Neurol 1921;27:82–95.

9 Seuntjens W: Gaap! De ontdekking van de geeuw. Eindhoven, De Boekenmakers, 2007.

10 Lelarge de Lignac JA: Examen serieux & comique des discours sur l'esprit. Part II. Amsterdam, s.e., 1759, p 461.

11 d'Arras G: Ille et Galeron (c. 1180). Paris, Champion, 1988, p 127.

12 Clark, DR: Stretching and Yawning with Yeats and Pound. The Malahat Review, 1974;29:104–17.

13 Nicoloff A: Bulgarian Folktales. Cleveland (OH), A. Nicoloff, 1979, pp 168–9.

14 Anderson JR, Myowa-Yamakoshi M, Matsuzawa T: Contagious yawning in chimpanzees. Proc Biol Sci. 2004;271(suppl 6):S468–S470.

15 Paukner A, Anderson JR: Video-induced yawning in stumptail macaques (Macaca arctoides). Biol Lett 2006;2:36–38.

16 Joly-Mascheroni RM, Senju A, Shepherd AJ: Dogs catch human yawns. Biol Lett 2008;4:446–448.

17 de Waal FBM: Putting the Altruism Back into Altruism: The Evolution of Empathy. Ann Rev Psychol 2008;59:279–300.

18 Portmann A: Animals as Social Beings. New York, Viking Press, 1961 [1953], p 213.

19 Lindsay SR: Handbook of Applied Dog Behavior and Training. (Volume III – Procedures and Protocols), Oxford, Blackwell, 2000, p 141.

20 Kraus K: Beim Wort genommen. Munich, Kösel-Verlag, 1955, p 432.

21 Goldie L, Green JM: Yawning and epilepsy. J Psychosom Res. 1961;5:263–268.

22 Muchnik S, Finkielman S, Semeniuk G, de Aguirre MI: Bostezo y epilepsia del lóbulo temporal. Medicina (B Aires) 2003;63:229–232.

23 Aull-Watschinger S, Pataraia E, Baumgartner C: Sexual auras: predominance of epileptic activity within the mesial temporal lobe. Epilepsy Behav 2008;12:124–127.

24 Udwadia ZF, Udwadia FE, Rao PP, Kapadia F: Penile hyperexcitability with recurrent ejaculations as the presenting manifestation of a case of rabies. Postgrad Med J 1988;64:85–86.

25 Beek HH: Waanzin in de middeleeuwen. Nijkerk (Netherlands), Callenbach, 1969, p 127.

26 Crenshaw TL, Goldberg JP: Sexual Pharmacology: Drugs That Affect Sexual Functioning. New York, W.W. Norton, 1996.

27 McLean JD, Forsythe RG, Kapkin IA: Unusual side effects of clomipramine associated with yawning. Can J Psychiatry 1983;28:569–570.
28 O'Brien CP: Drug addiction and drug abuse; in J. G. Hardman et al. (eds): The Goodman and Gilman's: The Pharmaceutical Basis of Therapeutics, ed 9. New York, McGraw Hill, 1996.
29 Kosztolányi D: 'Esti Kornél', in Összes novellái II. Budapest, Osiris Kiadó, 2007 [1933], p 473.
30 de Moor M: The Virtuoso. London, Picador, 1996 [1993], p 98.
31 Reber AS: The Penguin Dictionary of Psychology. Harmondsworth, Penguin, 1985, p 618.
32 Hardy T: The Hand of Ethelberta. London, Macmillan, 1912 [1876], p 74.

Wolter Seuntjens
J.-F. Leemanslaan 27
BE–1160 Oudergem Brussels (Belgium)
Tel. +32 2 6622 742
E-Mail seuntjens@baillement.com

Walusinski O (ed): The Mystery of Yawning in Physiology and Disease.
Front Neurol Neurosci. Basel, Karger, 2010, vol 28, pp 63–76

Non-Human Primates: A Comparative Developmental Perspective on Yawning

James R. Anderson

University of Stirling, Stirling, Scotland

Abstract

There is a long history of yawning in Old World monkeys being viewed as a form of communication, in particular, as a kind of threat. Yawning in agonistic and tense situations is seen in adult males, in particular, and it varies with male hormonal levels and social status. Experiments are reviewed that demonstrate operant control of the rate of yawning in adult male macaques, using food rewards. This indicates a degree of flexibility in the production of yawning. However, although adult male Old World monkeys often engage in 'canine contests', there is little evidence for the contagious yawning seen in humans. Experiments are reviewed showing that chimpanzees tested under comparable conditions to human adults, namely exposed to video sequences showing yawns, may yawn contagiously to yawn stimuli. Chimpanzees also yawn to computer animations of yawns. There is controversy in the literature over whether other species, including dogs and some monkeys, may also show contagious yawning. Further research is required to address unresolved issues. A hypothesis is put forward that in modern industrial society adults' natural pattern of yawning is inhibited, and that being reminded to yawn by seeing another individual yawn (contagious yawning) can help us to catch up on missed yawns. This would explain the lack of contagious yawning reported in young children and chimpanzees in natural surroundings, as these populations do not have the same social constraints on yawning.

Yawning as Communication

Yawning as a form of ritualized display in nonhuman primates was commented upon by Darwin [1], who described it as an expression of passion and anger in baboons and other Old World monkeys. Many observations of captive primates have supported this view. For example, Zuckerman [2] described 'bachelor' Hamadryas baboons about to engage in conflict as 'yawning' (he used inverted commas) in association with teeth grinding, grimacing and staring at the intended target of the aggression. Plate XVIII in Zuckerman [2] clearly shows yawning by an adult male baboon described as 'threatening'. Early field studies of Old World monkeys further added to the evidence for yawning as a form of communication. Remarking how yawning clearly displays the large canine teeth of adult males, Hall and DeVore [3] proposed a 'secondary intimidating effect' (p. 100) for this behavior in baboons. Those authors published two photographs showing the unworn canines of a young adult male baboon yawning 'under tension', and the broken and worn canine teeth of an old adult male yawning, respectively. Two more photographs in the same chapter describe adult males as 'harassing' other adult males, and in each case the harassing male is clearly yawning. Interestingly, in the same volume, Simonds [4] draws attention to the generally better condition of the canine teeth of dominant males in a wild group of bonnet macaques compared to more subordinate males, and he describes how serious wounding may occur during fights. Simonds [4] does not include yawning among the gestures used to determine dominance ranks within the group, but a photograph illustrating the well-developed canines of a fully adult male clearly shows the male yawning (p. 181). Laboratory analysis of the scanpaths of rhesus monkeys visually exploring photographs of conspecifics' faces provides good evidence for the 'canine display' aspect of yawning: when presented with photos of adult males yawning, around 50% of viewing monkeys' first saccades to the mouth were directed precisely to the canines, whereas photos of open-mouth threat elicited less specific saccades to the mouth area and to the ears [5].

Several lines of evidence link the frequency of yawning in adult male Old World monkeys to dominance rank. In sexually dimorphic polygynous species, such as macaques and baboons, there is a marked sex difference in the frequency of yawning: adult males easily out-yawn other age and sex classes [6]. In Celebes macaques, the rate of yawning by adult males varied with changes in their dominance status [7]. In wild olive baboons, the frequency of 'nondirected' yawning in the proximity of immigrant males varied with the condition of the displaying males' canines [8], and possibly reflected heightened tension. One adult male with broken canines refrained from yawning [8]. Bertrand [9] reported that only stumptail macaque males of high social rank responded by yawning when she looked at them; other males, over whom Bertand claimed to be dominant, showed no such response. She also noted teeth-grinding accompanying the dominant males' yawns, and characterized the latter as threat yawns, rather than tension yawns.

When individually housed adult male stumptail macaques were introduced into the same cage, dominant individuals showed more yawning than subordinates [10]. Those staged encounters gave rise to physical attacks; injurious aggression can be avoided while yawning rate is increased in experimental encounters between unfamiliar adult males separated by a transparent partition (rhesus macaques [11]). Adult males may also yawn prodigiously when confronted with their reflection in a mirror (e.g. various species of macaques [11, 12]and patas monkeys [11, 13]). Semifree-ranging adult male Barbary macaques yawned more just after triadic encounters involving an infant (sometimes referred to as 'agonistic buffering') than during the encounters. The only one of 7 studied males not to show this effect was the most dominant male in the group [14]. The authors suggested that yawning was actively inhibited during the male-male body contact phase of an encounter, and that physical separation between the males switched off the inhibitory effect and thereby permitted a 'tension component' to be expressed in the form of yawning.

Voluntary Control of Yawning by Adult Male Macaques

Information of the type reviewed in the previous section, specifically the fact that adult male Old World monkeys yawn readily in a range of situations characterized by tension or arousal, and that at least some yawns appears to be communicatory (note the distinction between 'directed' and 'undirected' yawns [6]), stimulated our first experimental studies of yawning in nonhuman primates. The question was whether adult male macaques could bring yawning under voluntary control. Although there was positive evidence for operant conditioning of a few naturally occurring behaviors in monkeys, such as vocalizations [15] and self-scratching [16], there were no previous attempts to train monkeys to produce yawns in order to obtain food rewards. Our first study used 2 behaviorally normal adult male pigtailed macaques housed in individual cages [17]. During 3 initial phases (each consisting of three 1-hour sessions), each monkey was passively observed by the experimenter, then given 20 pieces of fruit at random intervals during the session, then given fruit every time the facial expression 'protruded lips' was shown, respectively. Together these phases are referred to as condition A. There then followed 5 sessions in which all yawns were rewarded with a piece of fruit, handed to the monkey by the experimenter. This is condition B. In the first session of condition B, monkey 'Bernt' was trained to yawn through a procedure of successive approximations: at first any mouth-opening act was immediately followed by a reward. By the end of the first session, simply opening the mouth went unrewarded; instead only full yawns were reinforced, including full lip retraction, wide opening of the mouth, and a climatic tilting of the head upwards and backwards to expose the teeth. The second male, 'Charlie', was rewarded from the start of condition B only for producing full yawns.

Figure 1 shows the huge increase in yawning by both males in condition B (continuous reinforcement) compared to condition A (baseline). It is unclear whether the slight variation in procedure used with the 2 males (successive approximation vs. full yawn required from the outset) played a role in the higher rate of yawning produced by Bernt. Condition C consisted of 2 extinction sessions: no rewards were given; it is clear that both males' rate of yawning quickly diminished to baseline levels when no rewards were forthcoming. There then followed another session of continuous reinforcement, which saw yawn rates rise rapidly again (condition D). Finally, a closing extinction phase in which no rewards were given led to another decline in yawning to baseline levels (condition E).

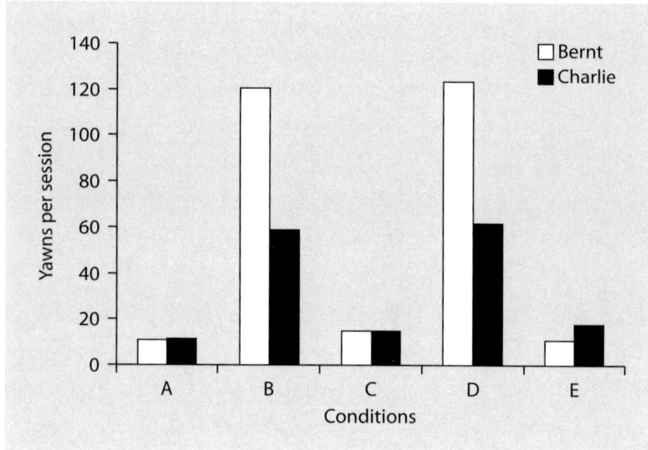

Fig. 1. Frequency of yawns produced by 2 adult male pig-tail macaques under different conditions of reinforcement. Conditions are as follows: A = baseline; B = continuous reinforcement; C = extinction; D = continuous reinforcement; E = extinction. After Louboungou and Anderson [17].

This study provided us with the first evidence that adult male macaques, like humans, could make themselves yawn. As described by Barbizet [18] for humans trying to make themselves yawn, Bernt and Charlie would open their mouths and appear to inhale deeply; both were also seen to abandon some attempts, further suggesting that they were deliberately trying to trigger yawns. These attempts were made while the monkey looked away from the experimenter. Upon successful completion of a yawn, the monkey would then orient towards the experimenter and sometimes extend a hand to receive the reward.

In a follow-up study, we used a similar procedure with 2 adult males of another species – tonkean macaques – with similar results [19]. Two new findings in this second study were: (1) a short-lived increase in yawning rates at the start of extinction sessions, reminiscent of the 'partial reinforcement effect' described in the learning literature, and (2) the especially high rates of yawning obtained when a fixed-ratio-3 reward contingency was used, i.e. a reward was given only after the monkey produced 3 yawns. This second study therefore confirmed that adult male macaques can voluntarily increase their rate of yawning when yawning is associated with obtaining rewards, and inhibit their rate of yawning when no extrinsic rewards are obtained.

One of the tonkean macaque males trained to yawn produced a mixture of 'slow' and 'fast' yawns during the experimental phases. Yawns of the latter type were also frequently produced when this male came into visual contact with his former group, and also when he was confronted with his mirror image [11]. Are fast and slow yawns functionally different? Several authors have made the distinction between yawns whose main function might be communication and those that are simply due to fatigue or boredom. For example, Zuckerman [2] noted that baboons yawned not just as a form of harassment but probably also '... in the human sense, from fatigue or boredom' (p. 262). He did not suggest differences in form between display and fatigue yawns, but various authors have invoked differences in the extent of teeth exposure, ear-flattening and eyebrow-raising, among other morphological aspects [e.g. 3, 9, 20]. Like humans, monkeys may show a peak in yawning shortly after wakening up [7, 21], and it would clearly be wrong to attribute a communicatory function to all yawns by adult males. Indeed, in his careful analysis of hundreds of yawns in groups of Old World monkeys, Deputte [21] concluded that around 90% of all yawns were 'rest' yawns, whereas only 10% could be described as 'emotion' or 'tension' yawns.

Voluntary Yawning: Some Implications and Questions

It would appear that even among Old World monkeys, most yawns are a consequence of states such as fatigue or drowsiness. Nevertheless, if even a subset of yawns can be used as a social signal, it would be useful for an individual to be able to control their production. Our two studies on operant conditioning of yawning in adult male macaques provided evidence of this ability, and raised a number of potentially interesting questions that mostly remain unanswered, such as:

– Is the capacity for voluntary production and inhibition of yawning limited to Old World monkeys, or does it also exist in other nonhuman primates? As mentioned previously, the studies conducted on operant conditioning of yawning specifically used adult male macaques because of their known propensity for yawning in a range of contexts. It would therefore be useful to extend this line of work to other species, including those with different species-typical social structures and degrees of sexual dimorphism in body size. For example, we would expect it to be quite easy to increase the rate of yawning by adult males of other polygynous Old World monkeys in which adult males are bigger than females, with greater canine development. One the other hand, gibbons – the so-called 'lesser apes' – are generally considered to be monogamous rather than polygynous, and there is much less of a difference in body size and in canine size between males and females than in the Cercopithecidae. Gibbons obviously yawn, but despite the lack of any detailed information on contexts of occurrence and frequency of yawning throughout the day, it seems safe to suggest that yawning in gibbons contains no element of threat. It is not even clear whether there is a sex difference in frequency of yawning (there does not appear to be any sex difference in human adults' rate of yawning either [22]). Can adult male or adult female gibbons exert voluntary control over their yawning? Nobody has attempted to find out.
– Can other age and sex classes control yawning? This question applies not just to Old World monkeys, but also to other species. For example, yawning rates in male macaques rise considerably with the onset of puberty, indicating a role for circulating androgens in preparedness to yawn [7, 23]. Castration of adult male rhesus almost totally eliminated yawning in a study of the effects of hormones on sexual behaviour; administration of testosterone reversed this effect [24].

Interestingly, administration of exogenous androgens increases the rate of yawning in adult female macaques to levels typical of adult males, whereas anti-androgen treatment blocks this effect [25, 26]. Such data indicate that, although under normal circumstances adult females yawn much less frequently than males, the requisite neural structures are in place that would allow flexible use of yawning by females. Of course, the development of the ability to control yawn production should also be amenable to study. Yawning clearly starts off as a reflex act; the question is at what point do individuals become able to (at least partly) overcome the reflexive aspect of the act and either voluntarily induce yawns, or inhibit them.

- One potentially interesting case to study might involve a species in which adult females are dominant over adult males. In the lemur branch of prosimian primates, for example, females are often, though not always, dominant over males [27]. Yawning occurs during agonistic interactions in ring-tailed lemurs; yawns that occurred during aggressive encounters including stink-fights were described as tension yawns [28]. They occurred mostly during pauses in the conflict, and were associated with displacement activities such as chewing movements and self-grooming. In other words, there is no evidence for yawns as displays in female lemurs, who in terms of body size are similar to adult males. When an unfamiliar adult female ringtail was introduced into a small captive group containing 2 males and an adult female, both females engaged in agonistic interactions, and both yawned repeatedly, particularly in the first few minutes of the introduction; the 2 males did not show aggression-related yawns [29]. It is not known whether yawning can be brought under operant control in lemurs of either sex.
- Can other species control the production of yawns? Concerning non-primates, only 1 study appears to have asked whether yawning rates can be manipulated through reinforcement schedules. It was reported that domestic dogs rewarded for yawning tended to produce 'pseudo-yawns', consisting of simply opening the mouth [30]. Dogs would be a particularly interesting species to study in this respect given the recent burgeoning literature claiming to demonstrate impressive social and cognitive achievements in these animals. Indeed, there now exists a claim and a counter-claim concerning whether dogs show contagious yawning after seeing a human yawn. Discussion of these studies will be deferred until later. Before then, we turn to the question of the contagiousness of yawning in primates.

Contagious Yawning

Although yawning may be ubiquitous across vertebrates, it has long been held that the phenomenon of contagious yawning is uniquely human [31, 32]. Although group-living species with highly synchronized behavioral profiles might show bouts of yawning at around the same time, such as upon awaking in the morning, or resting and digesting after feeding (e.g. lions [33]), the literature is remarkably lacking in descriptions of contagious yawning between nonhumans that are not explainable in terms of simple activity synchrony. Humans may see somebody yawning at any time of day, in any one of a wide variety of contexts, and be induced to yawn in turn. However, there is a huge range of both between- and within-individual differences in our susceptibility to contagious yawning. It is not an obligatory response; we do not yawn every time we see somebody else yawning, and in fact some people appear quite resilient to the effect (e.g. autistic children, when compared to typically developing children [34]). In experiments designed to assess susceptibility to contagious yawning, researchers usually ask people to watch controlled stimuli in the form of video images showing repeated yawning. Under these conditions, typically around 40–55% of participants (normal, young adults) report that they yawned [35, 36]. Investigation of factors underlying individual differences in this effect are still at a very early stage, but it would appear that people who score relatively highly on questionnaire measures of empathy and mental state attribution skills are more likely to yawn in response to seeing somebody else yawn [36].

The ease of constructing video sequences to show multiple examples of conspecifics yawning, and the knowledge that chimpanzees are capable of showing empathy and self-recognition, stimulated us to investigate contagious yawning in chimpanzees [37–38]. Two 'yawn' videotapes were prepared, each showing 10 short clips (6–8 s each, separated by blanks) of a chimpanzee yawning. One of these videotapes featured familiar chimpanzees from the same research centre where the study was conducted (Primate Research Institute, Kyoto University, Japan), while the second showed unfamiliar wild chimpanzees. The clips variously showed young infants, adult males and adult females yawning, either sitting or lying down. Two control videotapes were matched for general content, but instead of yawns they showed facial expressions such as grinning or threatening, or other mouth movements.

Six adult female chimpanzees, all members of a group with considerable experience of non-invasive behavioral experiments but with no previous experience of such video stimuli, were the participants. If they felt like doing so, they responded to an invitation by the experimenter to leave their group in the outside enclosure and move into a familiar experimental booth. They were thus tested individually, except for 3 of them who each brought along their 3-year-old juvenile. Each adult female was tested for 4 sessions, with 1 yawn and 1 control video being presented in each session, for a total of 2 exposures to each video. Following a 5-min baseline/habituation period, a 35-cm video monitor placed at floor level near one glass wall of the booth was switched on, and one of the videotapes was presented (duration: approximately 3 min). When the videotape ended, the monitor was switched off and a 3-min post-video observation period started. There then followed a 5-min distraction period, after which the second videotape was presented and followed by another post-video observation period. All occurrences of yawning by the chimpanzees were recorded in real time and verified by subsequent video analysis, as the chimpanzees' general behavior during video presentation and the post-video periods was videotaped.

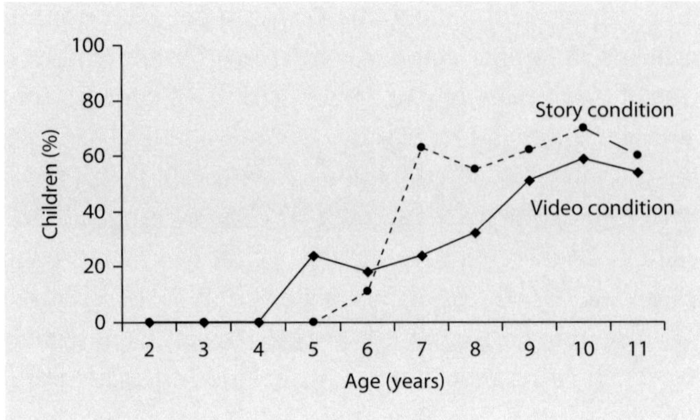

Fig. 2. Percentage of children at different ages showing yawning in response to seeing video yawns or to hearing or reading a story containing repeated references to yawning. After Anderson and Meno [39].

Two striking results emerged from this experiment. First, 2 of the females showed highly significant increases in yawning in response to yawn video stimuli compared to control stimuli; the 4 others showed no clear effects, always yawning relatively infrequently. So, in this small sample, 33% adult females showed contagious yawning. Although this is lower than the 40–50% of contagious yawners typically reported in studies with humans, in some ways the chimpanzee data can be seen as more impressive than the data from equivalent human studies. Note that human participants are usually instructed to self-monitor and report their yawns, and merely by thinking about their yawning, they are more likely to yawn. In contrast, apart from a general expectation about participating in some kind of task involving manipulating objects or a computer screen, the chimpanzees had no idea about why they were in the experimental booth; there was nothing to suggest to them that yawning was of some special interest. We therefore feel that contagious yawning in 33% of naïve naturally behaving chimpanzees compares favorably with data in humans.

The second striking outcome was that none of the 3 juveniles showed any yawning whatsoever during the study, in spite of watching yawns on the video monitor and also seeing their mothers yawn (one juvenile's mother was one of the 2 highly contagiously-yawning females described above). This finding is of interest in view of the finding that human children below the age of 5 years also appear to be immune to the yawn-inducing effects of yawns by other individuals [39]. Children ranging in age from 2 to 11 years were shown a video of an adult talking about a visit to the zoo and reciting nursery rhymes, and frequently breaking off to yawn. Direct observations of the children during exposure to the videotape and during post-video observations revealed an absence of yawning in preschoolers, and a subsequent gradual increase throughout childhood in the tendency to 'catch' another's yawn (fig. 2), reaching adult-like levels by the age of 11 or 12 years. In another condition, preschoolers were read a story in which the central character yawned repeatedly; older children read the book for themselves. The overall similarity of the results to those obtained in the video condition suggest that

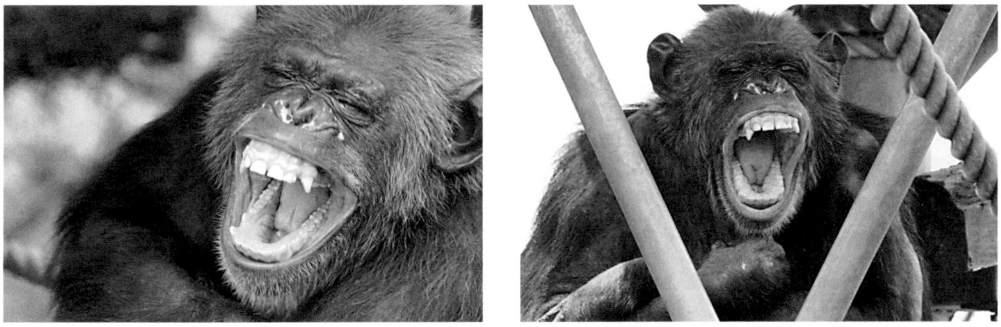

Fig. 3. Yawning in an adult female chimpanzee. Photos: T. Matsuzawa.

very young children are not vulnerable to 'psychological' inductors of yawning, such as seeing someone else yawn, or reading or thinking about yawning. Furthermore, the overall similarity between chimpanzees and humans in the effectiveness of video yawns for inducing yawning in adults, but not young juveniles, implies some commonality of mechanisms underlying the phenomenon of contagious yawning in humans and our nearest evolutionary neighbors. The cognitive correlates of contagious yawning in developing human and great ape children remain to be clarified.

Contagious Yawning: Recent Developments and Controversies

Another aspect of yawning in chimpanzees that indicates greater commonality with its human counterpart than with yawning in Old World monkeys is that it appears to serve no agonistic signaling function. Although chimpanzees may yawn due to tiredness, boredom, or mild tension or uncertainty, and show more than one type of yawn [40, 41] (fig. 3), there is no suggestion of anything like the 'canine contests' that occur in adult male macaques and baboons; this is in spite of the fact that chimpanzees show some degree of sexual dimorphism in body size and canine development. However, then it might be asked why, despite hundreds of thousands of hours of observations in the wild, in zoos and in laboratories, has nobody ever described naturally occurring contagious yawning in chimpanzees? One possibility is that it does occur in the wild, but at times of the day when humans are unlikely to see it occurring, such as immediately after waking early in the morning, while chimpanzees are in their arboreal nests, or at dusk, when chimpanzees are starting to settle in their nests for the night. An alternative possibility is that the phenomenon does not exist under natural circumstances in either wild or captive chimpanzees, or if it does, it is extremely rare. It may well be that video sequences showing sequences of yawns constitute a kind of supernormal stimulus that is able to trigger a contagious effect in some, though not all, chimpanzees.

Recent support for a 'supernormal stimulus'-induced contagious yawning effect in chimpanzees comes from a study involving presentation of computer-animated stimuli representing chimpanzees either yawning or displaying control mouth movements [42]. Two-dozen captive chimpanzees were tested, and on average they yawned over 2.5 times more frequently to the yawn animations than to control animations. Furthermore, it was established that the chimpanzees attended to the yawn and control animations for similar amounts of time; thus, ruling out differential saliency as a factor.

An obvious question is: if video stimuli can induce contagious yawning in chimpanzees even if they do not normally show the phenomenon, would the same happen for monkeys? As already described, 'canine contests' can involve two or more individuals yawning at around the same time, but there is no evidence that monkeys show true contagious yawning, rather than simply an escalation of a tension- or display-related behavior in adult male Old World monkeys. To conduct the only study so far to address this question [43], we prepared a video showing 10 naturally occurring yawns by members of a captive group of stumptail macaques; all yawns were considered to occur in relaxed, not tense situations. A control tape showed 10 facial actions such as those that occur during vocalizing, teeth-chattering or chewing. The 2 tapes were matched for general structure and total duration (1 min 30 s). The video stimuli were presented via a video monitor placed near a window so that any monkeys in the colony room could clearly see what was on the screen. The experimenter had an unobstructed view of all monkeys is the colony room, and recorded all occurrences of yawning during video presentation and for 3 min afterwards.

Over 14 yawn and 14 control sessions, every monkey except 1 adult female yawned at least once during at least 1 test session. Although there were no significant effects at the individual level, at group level, the average number of yawns in control sessions was 2.4 per individual, compared to 4.3 in yawn sessions, a significant difference. There was no overall relationship between dominance rank, sex or familiarity with the stimulus monkeys on yawning frequency.

So, does this finding of a group-level increase in yawning to the yawn video compared to the control video constitute evidence of contagious yawning in stumptail macaques? The evidence is not compelling, for a couple of reasons. First, as well as yawning more in the yawn condition, the monkeys also scratched themselves more; together, yawning and scratching can be a sign of anxiety or uncertainly. Second, over half of the yawns in the yawn video (6/10) were performed by an adult male. As already described, yawns by adult males draw attention to the canines, and can be interpreted as a kind of threat. Therefore, increased yawning accompanied by scratching in yawn video sessions might have been due to an increased feeling of uneasiness arising from seeing an adult male yawn repeatedly. In fact, 1 of the 2 adult males in the group was responsible for approximately half of all the yawns seen in the yawn condition. Our conclusion at present is that even with a 'supernormal stimulus' in the form of video yawn stimuli, there is not yet any strong evidence for contagious yawning in any species other than humans and chimpanzees.

Recently, however, this view has been challenged by a report of contagious yawning in gelada baboons [44]. Using data on over 3,000 yawns collected from a zoo-housed group of 21 individuals organized into 2 one-male units, it was shown that monkeys likely to have seen another individual yawning were more likely to yawn within a 5-min period than if the latter individual had not yawned. The effect appeared most strongly for adult females. Furthermore, 3 types of yawn were distinguished, called 'covered teeth', 'uncovered teeth' and 'uncovered gums', and the second individual to yawn was significantly more likely to produce the same type of yawn as the model, especially when the pair consisted of females. Finally, within 1 one-male unit (gelada social structure is based on subgroups containing 1 fully adult male and several adult females plus associated offspring), there was a positive correlation between frequency of grooming and temporal proximity of yawns between individuals. The authors interpreted the findings as follows: '... the matching response recorded between females probably reflects the need and ability of females to stay in tune with each others' behavioral activities and to form coalitions and alliances based on a precise reading of others behavior' (p. 4).

Clearly this report raises several questions that future research needs to address before gelada baboons can be admitted to the 'club of contagious yawners'. For example, what is the functional significance of the 3 different types of yawn (if any), and why should there be precise matching in contagion? What proportion of contagious yawns occurred between members belonging to different one-male units, as presumably these individuals are less empathic towards each other than those belonging to the same unit? Is it possible that the observed yawning in close temporal proximity indicates general behavioral synchrony of the type seen, for example, in lions, rather than true contagious yawning? Why has contagious yawning never been reported in other primate species in which bonds among females (including members of the same matriline) are crucially important?

It is not just in primates that yawning gives rise to controversy. Reflecting the growing wave of new research investigating the social and cognitive abilities of domestic dogs, one recent report claimed that dogs yawned when they observed a human yawning, but not when the human made control (non-yawn) mouth movements [45]. The size of the effect was impressive, with 21 of 29 dogs tested showing a positive response; indeed this percentage (72%) is considerably higher than the corresponding value in studies with humans (45–60%), although the latter studies usually use video models rather than a live model. This apparent cross-species contagion effect was attributed to dogs' advanced capacity for empathy, with the suggestion that it might help 'coordinate dog-human interaction and communication' (p. 446); the paper received considerable media coverage. There are, however, several issues that call for prudence before accepting this study as evidence of cross-species contagious yawning by dogs. For example, in the 'yawn' condition, after attracting the dog's attention the experimenter started to simulate yawning accompanied by vocalizations (the nature of the vocalizations is not described); these yawn-vocalization pairings were presented 10–19 times over a 5-min period. In the control condition, non-yawn mouth movements were made, but without vocalizations, and it is unclear whether the frequency of repetitions was matched with that in the experimental condition. It therefore seems possible that the particularly strange behavior of the experimenter in the yawn condition, consisting of repeated yawning movements and vocalizations, caused a state of unease or anxiety in the dogs, giving rise to yawning.

Indeed, another study using controlled video sequences showing humans and dogs yawning or making control mouth movements obtained no strong evidence that dogs 'catch' yawns either of humans or conspecifics [46]. Only 1 of 15 dogs tested showed significantly more yawns during yawn videos (5 yawns in total) than during the open-mouth (0 yawns), and even that, the authors point out, could have arisen by chance. It should be obvious that the question of contagious yawning in dogs requires further study before concluding that they might show an even greater effect than humans.

Concluding Comments

Hopefully, this review of some of the comparative literature on yawning will stimulate further interest in the phenomenon not only in humans, but in nonhumans too. It is clear that we have a lot more to learn about the psychological influences on yawning, how this varies during development, and what the implications are for individuals' social and self-awareness. To conclude, I will offer some thoughts relevant to the intriguing question: 'Why does contagious yawning exist?' Consider the following: as other chapters in this book show, yawning gives rise to a suite of physiological changes (e.g. in cortical temperature, oxygen uptake and CO_2 dispersal, inner ear pressure equalization). Under normal conditions, these changes are beneficial to the organism. However, in many human societies it is considered impolite to yawn in the presence of others [47]. I suggest that inhibition of yawning due to social pressures and other factors such as a busy working life actually gives rise to a kind of yawn deprivation in many people. In other words, we 'forget' to yawn as much as we should, or at least when we normally should. It may therefore be that by virtue of a low-level empathic processes, seeing (or hearing) somebody else yawn, or reading or thinking about yawning, might function to remind our brain that it might be a good idea to yawn, which in turn will lead to some of the beneficial physiological effects outlined above. From this perspective, the lack of contagious yawning in young children becomes easier to explain, as youngsters do not have the same degree of inhibition when it comes to yawning in public. Young children yawn wherever and whenever they feel like it, which is usually when they are tired. Likewise, chimpanzees do not have the same kinds of social constraints on yawning as human adults do; they appear to be liberated yawners [e.g. 41]. Chimpanzees are capable of showing empathy with other individuals, but because under normal circumstances they have little need to catch up on yawning, they show little susceptibility to the contagious yawning effect that we see in human adults. It is only when some form of extra yawning stimulation is given to chimpanzees, for example in the form of repeated video or animated images, that they may be moved to show the effect.

References

1 Darwin C: The Expression of Emotions in Man and Animals (1872). Chicago, University of Chicago, 1965.

2 Zuckerman S: The Social Life of Monkeys and Apes. London, Kegan Paul, Trench, Trubner & Co., 1932.

3 Hall KRL, DeVore I: Baboon social behavior; in DeVore I (ed): Primate Behavior: Field Studies of Monkeys and Apes. New York, Holt, Rinehart and Winston, 1965, pp 53–110.

4 Simonds PE: The bonnet macaque in south India; in DeVore I (ed): Primate Behavior: Field Studies of Monkeys and Apes. New York, Holt, Rinehart and Winston, 1965, pp 175–196.

5 Gothard KM, Erickson CA, Amaral DG: How do rhesus monkeys (*Macaca mulatta*) scan faces in a visual paired comparison task? Anim Cogn 2004; 7:25–36.

6 Redican WK: Facial expressions in nonhuman primates; in Rosenblum LA (ed): Primate Behavior: Developments in Field and Laboratory Research. New York, Academic Press, 1975, vol 4, pp 103–194.

7 Hadidian J: Yawning in an Old World monkey (*Macaca nigra*). Behaviour 1980;75:133–147.

8 Packer C: Male dominance and reproductive activity in *Papio anubis*. Anim Behav 1979;27:37–45.

9 Bertrand M: The Behavioral Repertoire of the Stumptail Macaque. Basel, Karger, 1969.

10 Adams DB, Schoel WM: A statistical analysis of the social behavior of the male stumptail macaque (*Macaca arctoides*). Am J Primatol 1982;2:249–273.

11 Anderson JR: Self-Recognition in Primates: Experiments with Mirrors. 16 mm film, VHS and DVD. Goettingen, Institut für den Wissenschaftlichen Film, 1997 (34.5 min).

12 Anderson JR: The Face in the Mirror. VHS. Paris, Leo Productions, 1995.

13 Hall KRL: Behaviour of monkeys towards mirror images. Nature 1962;196:1258–1261.

14 Roshani A, Todt D, Janik VM, Hultsch H: Yawning in male Barbary macaques (*Macaca sylvanus*); in Roeder JJ, Thierry B, Anderson JR, Herrenschmidt N (eds): Current Primatology. Strasbourg: Université Louis Pasteur, 1994, vol 2: Social Development, Learning and Behaviour, pp 81–86.

15 Pierce JD: A review of attempts to operantly condition alloprimate vocalization. Primates 1985;26:202–213.

16 Iversen IH, Ragnarsdottir GA, Randrup KI: Operant conditioning of autogrooming in vervet monkeys (*Cercopithecus aethiops*). J Exp Anal Behav 1984;42: 171–189.

17 Louboungou M, Anderson JR: Yawning, scratching, and protruded lips: differential conditionability of natural acts in pigtail monkeys (*Macaca nemestrina*). Primates 1987;28:367–375.

18 Barbizet J: Yawning. J Neurol Neurosurg Psychiat 1958;21:203–209.

19 Anderson JR, Wunderlich D: Food-reinforced yawning in *Macaca tonkeana*. Am J Primatol 1988; 16:165–169.

20 Anderson JR, McGrew WC: Guinea baboons (*Papio papio*) at a sleeping site. Am J Primatol 1984;6:1–14.

21 Deputte BL: Ethological study of yawning in primates. 1. Quantitative analysis and study of causation in two species of Old World monkeys (*Cercocebus albigena* and *Macaca fascicularis*). Ethology 1994;98: 221–245.

22 Schino G, Aureli F: Do men yawn more than women? Ethol Sociobiol 1989;10:375–378.

23 Troisi A, Aureli F, Schino G, Rinaldi F, de Angelis N: The influence of age, sex, and rank on yawning behavior in two species of macaques (*Macaca fascicularis* and *Macaca fuscata*). Ethology 1990;86: 303–310.

24 Phoenix CH, Slob AK, Goy RW: Effects of castration and replacement therapy on sexual behavior of adult male rhesuses. J Comp Physiol Psychol 1973; 84:472–481.
25 Goy RW, Resko JA: Gonadal hormones and behavior of normal and pseudohermaphroditic nonhuman female primates. Recent Prog Horm Res 1972; 28:707–733.
26 Graves FC, Wallen K: Androgen-induced yawning in rhesus monkey females is reversed with a nonsteroidal anti-androgen. Horm Behav 2006;49;233–236.
27 Pereira ME, Kaufman R, Kappeler PM, Overdorff DJ: Female dominance does not characterize all the Lemuridae. Folia Primatol 1990;55:96–103.
28 Jolly A: Lemur Behavior. Chicago, University of Chicago Press, 1966.
29 Roeder JJ, Fornasieri I, Anderson JR: Yawning in ringtailed lemurs (*Lemur catta*); in Roeder JJ, Thierry B, Anderson JR, Herrenschmidt N (eds): Current Primatology. Strasbourg, Université Louis Pasteur, 1994, vol 2: Social Development, Learning and Behaviour, pp 77–80.
30 Konorski J: Integrative Activity of the Brain: An Interdisciplinary Approach. Chicago, University of Chicago Press, 1967.
31 Lehmann HE: Yawning: a homeostatic reflex and its psychological significance. Bull Meninger Clin 1979;43:123–136.
32 Walusinski O: Baillements et Pandiculations. Brou, Oscitatio, 2004.
33 McKenzie AA: The tonsillar evacuation hypothesis of yawning behaviour. S Afr J Sci 1994;90:64–66.
34 Senju A, Maeda M, Kikuchi Y, Hasegawa T, Tojo Y, Osanai H: Absence of contagious yawning in children with autism spectrum disorder. Biol Lett 2007; 3:706–708.
35 Provine RR: Yawning as a stereotyped action pattern and releasing stimulus. Ethology 1986;72:448–455.
36 Platek SM, Critton SR, Myers TE, Gallup GG Jr: Contagious yawning: the role of self-awareness and mental state attribution. Cogn Brain Res 2003;17: 223–227.
37 Anderson JR, Myowa-Yamakoshi M, Matsuzawa T: Contagious yawning in chimpanzees. Proc R Soc Lond B 2004;271:S468–S470.
38 Anderson JR, Matsuzawa T: Yawning: an opening into empathy? in Matsuzawa T, Tomonga M, Tanaka M (eds): Cognitive Development in Chimpanzees. Tokyo, Springer, 2006, pp 233–245.
39 Anderson JR, Meno P: Psychological influences on yawning in children. Curr Psychol Lett: Behav Brain Cogn 2003;11:2. http://cpl.revues.org/document390.html.
40 Van Lawick-Goodall J: The behaviour of free-living chimpanzees in the Gombe Stream Reserve. Anim Behav Monogr 1968;1:161–311.
41 Vick S-J, Paukner A: Variation and context of yawns in captive chimpanzees (*Pan troglodytes*). Am J Primatol 2009, in press.
42 Campbell MW, Carter JD, Proctor D, Eisenberg ML, de Waal FBM: Computer animations stimulate contagious yawning in chimpanzees. Proc R Soc Lond B 2009;276:4255–4259.
43 Paukner A, Anderson JR: Video-induced yawning in stumptail macaques (*Macaca arctoides*). Biol Lett 2006;2:36–38.
44 Palagi E, Leone A, Mancini G, Ferrari PF: Contagious yawning in gelada baboons as a possible expression of empathy. Proc Natl Acad Sci USA 2009;106: 19262–19267.
45 Joly-Mascheroni RM, Senju A, Sheperd AJ: Dogs catch human yawns. Biol Lett 2008;4:446–448.
46 Harr AL, Gilbert VR, Phillips KA: Do dogs (*Canis familiaris*) show contagious yawning? Anim Cogn 2009;12:833–837.
47 Seuntjens W: On Yawning or The Hidden Sexuality of the Human Yawn; PhD Dissertation, Vrije Universiteit, Amsterdam, 2004, Brou/Veghel, Editions Oscitatio, 2004.

James R. Anderson
Department of Psychology, University of Stirling
Stirling FK9 4LA (Scotland)
Tel. +44 1786 46 76 37, Fax +44 1786 46 76 41
E-Mail jra1@stir.ac.uk

Walusinski O (ed): The Mystery of Yawning in Physiology and Disease.
Front Neurol Neurosci. Basel, Karger, 2010, vol 28, pp 77–83

Punishment-Induced Fear Modifies the Daily Course of Yawning in Rats

Alejandro Moyaho · Jaime Valencia

Laboratorio de Ecología de la Conducta, Instituto de Fisiología, Benemérita Universidad Autónoma de Puebla, Puebla, México

Abstract

A challenge in the study of yawning behavior is understanding the way external factors may modify it. This study investigated whether response-dependent punishment or random punishment decreased yawning by the application of buzzer noise paired with electric shocks in a high-yawning strain of Sprague-Dawley male rats. Yawn rate increased daily in response to the experimental cage, and also to the buzzer noise. Two alternate periods of no punishment and punishment were followed by a final period of buzzer noise occurring alone. Punishment did not diminish yawning significantly in either condition although the yawn rate increased in the following period of no punishment and in the buzzer-noise period, relative to the period of yawn-dependent punishment. Yawn rate increased in the buzzer-noise period relative to the first period of no punishment and first period of random punishment. These findings indicate that there are constraints that impede the suppression of yawning using punishment, and that yawning is a delayed response to fear produced by response-dependent punishment.

Yawning is seen as a stereotypical action pattern [1] because no environmental input changes the sequence of participating movements, although yawning frequency could be modifiable. There is evidence indicating that this is so, at least in pigtail macaques, specifically *Macaca nemestrina* [2] and *Macaca tonkeana* [3], primate species in which the yawn rate increases using instrumental procedures. The opposite, a reduction in yawning frequency, has not been empirically studied [however, please see: 4]; nevertheless, it is known that social factors may inhibit overt yawning, though the motor pattern may still occur.

Contexts in which yawning occurs are varied, ranging from those where a subject is relaxed and/or probably bored [5], through embarrassing social situations, to those which produce anxiety, such as when a person waits for an important appointment [6]. Yawning is often associated with emotional situations, but these comprise a variable number of emotions [7]. Two of them, fear and anxiety, could have been confused in some studies on yawning [e.g. 8]. Fear, a reaction to a dangerous situation which is already real and well defined, differs from anxiety which is the emotional anticipation of an aversive situation difficult to predict and control [7].

In this study, we used a strain of Sprague-Dawley rats that yawns at a high rate (22 yawns/h [9]) and instrumental procedures to investigate: (1) whether yawning behavior can be diminished by punishing it with electric shocks, and (2) whether yawning is a response to fear or anxiety using response-dependent punishment and random punishment, respectively. In addition, we paired an auditory stimulus to the electric shock to see if rats associate one stimulus with the other.

Material and Methods

Study Subjects
Thirty-one high-yawning (HY) male rats were used at the age of 2 months. Rats were housed 4 per Acrylic cage (46 × 32 × 20 cm) with commercially available food and water provided at libitum, and maintained on a light-dark cycle (light: 07:00–19:00 h), and ambient temperature.

The HY strain was obtained by recording yawning in a sample of 2-month-old male rats, from which the male with the most yawns was crossed with one of his sisters. Then he was crossed with one of his daughters and afterwards the HY strain was maintained by brother-sister mating, selecting HY rats [9].

Experimental Apparatus
Yawning behavior was recorded in an experimental cage consisting of a glass cage (21 × 24 × 36 cm) that was open on the top and bottom and placed on a grid floor made of stainless steel rods (1-mm diameter and spaced at 1-cm intervals). Electric shocks (0.6–1.3 mA, 0.5 s) were delivered to the floor by an electric shock generator (60-Hz AC) made at the School of Electronics at the Benemérita Universidad Autónoma de Puebla. A digital multimeter was used to verify the intensity of the shocks on the floor rods. The experimental cage and the grid floor were cleaned before testing each rat. For the auditory stimulus, we used a buzzer (5-cm diameter, 80 dB) which was attached to a wood cage (36 cm high) placed next to the experimental cage. The buzzer was operated manually using a switch and chronometer.

Experimental Procedure
On days of the experiment, a trial started when rats were put singly into the experimental cage, which was on a table in a small room that was illuminated artificially. Yawning frequency was recorded to the nearest minute using a chronometer for 30 min on consecutive days from 14:00 to 16:00 h by 2 observers seated on opposite sides of the table. A yawn was considered as a slow opening of the mouth with inhaling and a more rapid closing and exhaling [10]. One group of 8 rats was observed and yawning recorded for 9 consecutive days with no additional stimulus other than that represented by the experimental cage. Another group of 8 rats was observed and its yawning recorded during 8 consecutive days. The first 3 days the rats received no additional stimulus other than that represented by the experimental cage, but the last 5 days they were presented with 7 buzzer noises (80 dB, 5 s) randomly delivered (for which a table of random numbers was used).

Punishment of yawning behavior consisted of delivering a 80-dB loud buzzer noise for 5 s, paired with an electric shock on the last 0.5 s and according to 2 experimental conditions: (1) Eight

Fig. 1. Daily course of yawn rate of HY adult male rats (n = 8). The boxes represent the distribution of yawning with a statistically significant difference between the first and last days (p = 0.001). Points represent means ± SE.

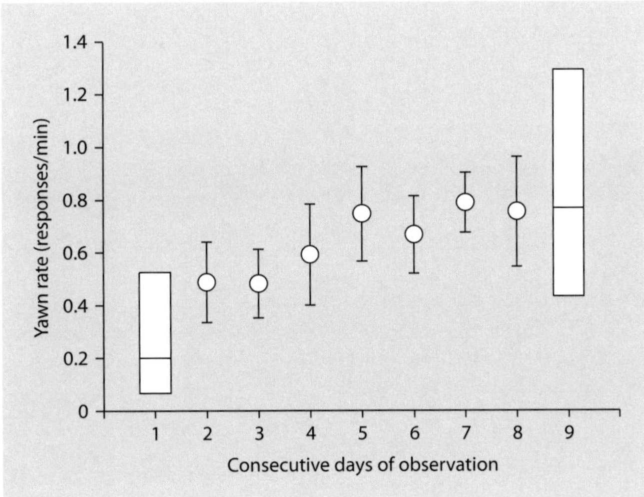

rats were observed and yawning recorded during 20 consecutive days. The occurrence of a cumulative number of yawns was followed by a buzzer noise paired with a foot shock. The number represented 20% of the yawning frequency attained the preceding period without buzzer-shock pairings, and was proportionally distributed during the 30 min of observation. In addition, the intensity of the electric shock was increased stepwise at 10-min intervals if yawn frequency surpassed the fixed upper limit of 20%. The intensity of the electric shock was increased to achieve a greater suppression of responding [11]. The buzzer-shock pairings were given over 5 and 4 consecutive days, each period preceded by 3-day periods without punishment, and followed by a 5-day period in which the buzzer noise alone occurred at 30-second intervals. (2) As above, but using 7 rats and with the buzzer-shock pairings delivered randomly.

Statistical Analysis

The yawn rate of each rat was pooled and averaged for each treatment (i.e. days in which either no punishment or buzzer-shock pairings or buzzer noise alone was applied to rats). A repeated-measures ANOVA was used to test for differences amongst treatments and Tukey's HSD test was used to make unplanned comparisons. The data were transformed whenever they did not comply with normality. A logistic regression [12] of the probability of yawn occurrence to the periods of punishment and no punishment together was applied to compare yawn course between response-dependent punishment and random punishment. The average yawn rate of the first period of no punishment served as a reference from which each rat's yawn rate was scored as 1 (above average) or 0 (below average). Exact p values are presented for the reader to assess the strength of the statistical results.

Results

Rats which were put in the experimental cage daily, with no stimulus other than the cage itself, had significantly increased their yawn rate on the last observation day (i.e.

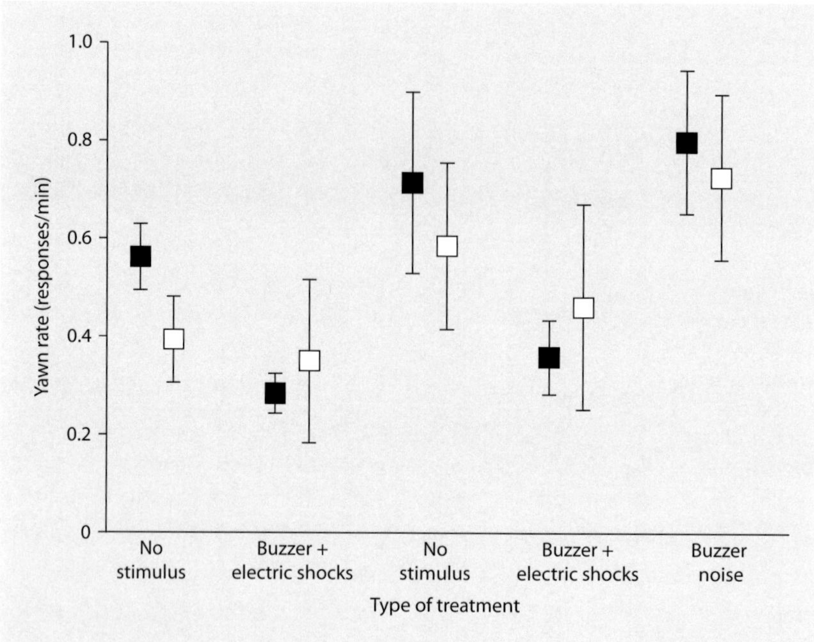

Fig. 2. The effect of buzzer noise paired with foot shocks on the rate of yawns (means ± SE) for 7–8 HY male rats. ■ = Buzzer-shock pairings contingent upon a cumulative number of yawns. The second period of no punishment and the period of buzzer noise alone are different from the corresponding first period of buzzer-shock pairings ($p = 0.022$ and $p = 0.004$, respectively). The period of buzzer noise alone is different from the second period of buzzer-shock pairings ($p = 0.019$). □ = Shock-buzzer pairings randomly delivered. The period of buzzer noise alone is different from the first period of no punishment ($p = 0.012$) and from the first period of randomly delivered buzzer-shock pairings ($p = 0.004$).

day 9) relative to day 1 (paired t test, $t_8 = 5.87$, $p = 0.001$; fig. 1). Yawn rate of rats which were presented with a random buzzer noise for 5 consecutive days did not differ from the preceding 3 days when no stimulus was added to the experimental cage (paired t test, $t_8 = 1.64$, $p = 0.146$).

ANOVA revealed significant differences amongst the treatments when yawns were followed by buzzer-shock pairings ($F_{4, 28} = 5.62$, $p = 0.002$; fig. 2). The post hoc analysis showed that yawn rate increased in the second period of no punishment ($p = 0.022$) and the period in which the buzzer noise alone was applied ($p = 0.004$) relative to the first period of buzzer-shock pairings. Yawning increased in the period in which only the buzzer noise was applied relative to the second period of buzzer-shock pairings ($p = 0.019$).

ANOVA also showed significant differences amongst treatments ($F_{4, 24} = 5.41$, $p = 0.003$; fig. 2) when the buzzer-shock pairings were randomly applied to the rats. Yawn rate in the period of buzzer noise alone was greater than in the first period of no punishment ($p = 0.012$) and the first period of buzzer-shock pairings ($p = 0.004$).

Table 1. The odds ratio for consecutive days of observation fitting a logistic regression model to yawn rate of HY rats

	First period of punishment + period of no punishment		Second period of punishment + period of buzzer noise alone	
	Yawn-dependent	Random	Yawn-dependent	Random
Odds ratio	2.85	1.46	1.53	1.3
95% CI	1.59–5.13	1.10–1.94	1.22–1.93	1.05–1.61

The odds ratio for days of the first period of punishment and second period of no punishment was higher for yawn-dependent punishment than for random punishment (table 1), although the difference was not significant. The odds ratio for days of the second period of punishment and the period of buzzer noise was also higher for yawn-dependent punishment than random punishment, but the difference was far from being significant (table 1).

Discussion

The main purpose of this study was to investigate how yawning frequency is affected when male adult rats are exposed to foot shocks in either of 2 conditions: response-dependent punishment or response-independent punishment given at random. Both conditions are expected to distinguish between fear and anxiety, respectively. Secondarily, a buzzer noise was paired with the foot shocks to determine if it lowered yawning frequency as a consequence of the possible association made by the rats between the two types of stimuli. Such association did not occur suggesting that conditioning of yawning, as other stereotyped behaviors, is unlikely.

Since repetitive exposure to the same test situation (e.g. an experimental cage) makes rats settle down, the increase in the overall rate of yawning from the first to the last observation day in the cage suggests that it is associated with relaxation or tranquility. So, as previously noted [13], an increase in yawning frequency seems to be correlated with a decreasing level of stress. However, in this study, when the rats were presented with buzzer noises and hence aroused, yawning frequency did not change and instead followed the daily course of increments. Therefore, the rats either habituated very quickly to the presence of the noises, which is unlikely, or there is a tendency for yawning to increase in response to mild stress [14]. An attempt to maintain arousal cannot be, as suggested by earlier studies [15], a satisfactory explanation as a random loud buzzer noise is already a disturbing stimulus.

The findings indicate that neither of the punishment regimes significantly diminished yawning frequency. This accords with previous studies where the difficulty of preventing [4] or increasing yawning frequency using positive reinforcement procedures was demonstrated [16]. The findings showed that response-dependent punishment prevents yawning from attaining the graded increase which characterizes daily exposure to the same test situation, while random punishment does not modify it. Random buzzer-shock pairings increased yawn rate in the buzzer noise condition relative to the first period of no punishment, and hence resembled what occurred when no aversive stimulus was present; however, yawn-dependent buzzer-shock pairings did not increase the rate. This difference indicates that fear caused by punishing yawning kept the overall rate of responding across testing days constant, although the moderate diminution due to punishment sufficed to reveal that yawning is a delayed response to fear. Anxiety produced by random buzzer-shock pairings, in contrast, did not change the constant increase in yawning throughout the testing days, suggesting that yawning is, in this study, insensitive to random presentation of aversive stimuli.

In summary, yawning is a delayed response to fear produced by response-dependent punishment, and is insensitive to anxiety produced by intermittent punishment. Further experiments will clarify the precise mechanisms whereby rats respond yawning to emotional conditions.

Acknowledgments

We thank Jochabert Rendón for her help in recording the yawning, and Alejandro Godinez for building the apparatus for electric shocks.

References

1 Provine RR, Hamernik HB: Yawning: effects of stimulus interest. Bull Psychonomic Soc 1986;24:437–438.
2 Louboungou M, Anderson JR: Yawning, scratching, and protruded lips: differential conditionability of natural acts in pigtail monkeys (*Macaca nemestrina*). Primates 1987;28:367–375.
3 Anderson JR, Wunderlich D: Food-reinforced yawning in *Macaca tonkeana*. Am J Primatol 1988; 16:165–169.
4 Greco M: Yawning facilitates the transition from lower to higher levels of arousal; doctoral dissertation, Philadelphia, Temple University, 1992.
5 Gallup AC, Gallup GG: Yawning and thermoregulation. Physiol Behav 2008;95:10–16.
6 Shader RI, Greenblatt DJ: Yawning and anxiety modulation. J Clin Psychopharmacol 1985;5:1.
7 Ramos A, Mormede P: Stress and emotionality: a multidimensional and genetic approach. Neurosci Biobehav Rev 1998;22:33–57.
8 Tufik S, Nathan CL, Neumann B, Hipólide DC, Lobo LL, de Medeiros R, Troncone LRP, Braz S, Suchecki D: Effects of stress on drug-induced yawning: constant vs. intermittent stress. Physiol Behav 1995;58:181–184.
9 Urbá-Holmgren R, Trucios N, Holmgren B, Eguibar JR, Gavito A, Cruz G, Santos A: Genotypic dependency of spontaneous yawning frequency in the rat. Behav Brain Res 1990;40:29–35.
10 Barbizet J: Yawning. J Neurol Neurosurg Psychiatry 1958;21:203–209.
11 Fantino EJ, Logan CA: The Experimental Analysis of Behavior: A Biological Perspective. New York, WH Freeman, 1979.

12 Quinn GP, Keough MJ: Experimental Design and Data Analysis for Biologists. Cambridge, Cambridge University Press, 2003.
13 Dourish CT, Cooper SJ: Neural basis of drug-induced yawning; in Cooper SJ, Dourish CT (eds): Neurobiology of Stereotyped Behaviour. Oxford, Clarendon Press, 1990, pp 91–116.
14 Moyaho A, Valencia J: Grooming and yawning trace adjustment to unfamiliar environments in laboratory Sprague-Dawley rats (*Rattus norvegicus*). J Comp Psychol 2002;116:263–269.
15 Baenninger M: On yawning and its functions. Psychonomic Bull Rev 1997;4:198–207.
16 Konorski J: Integrative Activity of the Brain. Chicago, University of Chicago Press, 1967.

Alejandro Moyaho
Laboratorio de Ecología de la Conducta, Instituto de Fisiología
Benemérita Universidad Autónoma de Puebla
Apartado Postal 406, Puebla, Pue. 72401 (México)
Tel. +52 222 229 5500, ext. 7306, Fax +52 222 229 5500, ext. 7301, E-Mail almoyaho@siu.buap.mx

Walusinski O (ed): The Mystery of Yawning in Physiology and Disease.
Front Neurol Neurosci. Basel, Karger, 2010, vol 28, pp 84–89

A Thermoregulatory Behavior

Andrew C. Gallup

Department of Biological Sciences, Binghamton University, Binghamton, N.Y., USA

Abstract

The existence of yawning across vertebrate species suggests important basic functions, and the spontaneous and involuntary nature of a yawn lends support for it having adaptive significance. Recent research suggests the biological function of yawning among homeotherms is central thermoregulation. Comparative research from birds, rats and humans shows that yawning reduces brain and body temperature, is influenced by the range and direction of ambient temperature change, and is inhibited by methods of behavioral cooling. This research provides strong support for the view that yawning stimulates or facilitates cortical arousal, demonstrating that a yawn is a behavioral response to transient brain hyperthermia, acting to counter intermittent increases in brain temperature and promote thermal homeostasis. This theory is powerful because it not only integrates a great deal of seemingly diverse information about yawning, but it can also be used to generate numerous testable predictions. Applications from this research range from basic physiological understanding to the improved treatment and understanding of diseases associated with thermoregulatory dysfunction.

Yawning is characterized by a large gaping of the mouth and eye closure, accompanied by a deep inhalation of air and a shorter expiration. Phylogenetically old, yawning has been documented in all 5 classes of vertebrates, suggesting it has important basic functions [1]. Although the mere occurrence of yawning across species is not evidence that it is an evolved adaptation, the spontaneous and involuntary nature of yawning lends support for its adaptive significance. Likewise, similar to other adaptive responses such as sneezing, yawning provides a brief sense of gratification in healthy populations [2]. To this point, however, attempts to identify the functional and primitive significance of yawning have led to little consensus [3].

One of the more widespread hypotheses attempting to explain the physiological purpose of yawning posits a role in respiration. In particular, a commonly held view is that yawning functions to equilibrate oxygen levels in the blood; however, this hypothesis remains unsupported. Provine et al. [4] showed that while breathing heightened levels of oxygen or carbon dioxide increased breathing rates, it did not influence yawning [4]. They also demonstrated that physical exercise sufficient to double breathing rates has no effect on yawning. Therefore, contrary to popular belief, it has been concluded that yawning does not serve a respiratory function, and that yawning and breathing are controlled by separate mechanisms.

Baenninger [5] has reviewed a vast amount of literature that suggests yawning functions to stimulate or facilitate arousal during state change. In line with this hypothesis, yawning occurs in anticipation of important events and during behavioral transitions or changes in activity levels across vertebrate taxa. Accordingly, it has been proposed that the adaptive function of yawning is to modify levels of cortical arousal. However, while this account may explain the hedonic quality and unprompted nature of yawning, the particular physiological mechanism for achieving such arousal has not been identified. Here, this chapter will describe the most recent empirical evidence indicating a role of yawning in central thermoregulation.

'Brain Cooling Hypothesis'

Brain temperature is determined by a number of variables, including the temperature of the blood supplying the brain, rate of blood flow through the brain, and rate of metabolic heat production. Cooling mechanisms include increased circulation, vasodilation, convection and conduction processes, heat dissipation through the upper airways, and the presence of venous plexuses or intertwined venous and arterial rete structures [6]. Recent research suggests/supports that yawning is involved in central thermoregulation [7–9]. According to this hypothesis, spontaneous yawning is triggered in response to mild central hyperthermia, acting to counter intermittent increases in brain temperature and promote thermal homeostasis. Thus, it is proposed that a yawn increases arousal and mental efficiency by maintaining optimal brain temperature.

It is well known that most instances of yawning tend to occur shortly after awakening and before sleeping [10, 11]. Body temperature begins to peak in the evening and the onset of sleep initiates a decline in core body temperature. Likewise, the tendency to wake-up occurs in tandem with a rise in core body temperature in the morning. Therefore consistent with the brain cooling hypothesis, yawning frequently occurs in the evening, when brain temperature is at its peak, and upon waking, when brain temperature begins increasing from its lowest point [12]. Yawning in early morning may be a compensatory thermal stabilizing mechanism. Waking disrupts a relaxed state, and rapid increases in movement and conscious brain activity produce ensuing metabolic increases in temperature. By lowering brain temperature and maintaining thermal homeostasis, this theory suggests that instead of prompting sleep, yawning actually serves to maintain focus and attention, thereby antagonizing sleep [7]. Furthermore, prolonged sleep deprivation in rats has been shown to increase deep brain temperature [13]. Subjective ratings of sleepiness in humans correlate with increases in skin temperature while lying down [14], and with increases in core body temperature when standing [15]. In addition, hot water consumption has been shown to increase body temperature as well as sleepiness, while ice intake produces the converse [16]. Therefore, it appears that variations in body temperature are associated with corresponding variations in sleepiness, and this may explain why people often yawn when they are tired [11].

Pharmacological research has demonstrated that yawning is under the control of the hypothalamus [17], and structures of the hypothalamus have been strongly linked to thermoregulation [18]. In support of the brain cooling hypothesis, the physiological consequences of a yawn are in accord with those that would be necessary for cerebral cooling [7, 8]. For instance, the deep inhalation of air taken into the lungs causes an acceleration in heart rate [19, 20] and also raises blood pressure [21]. More specifically, the constriction and relaxation of facial muscles during a yawn increases facial blood flow, and these changes are thought to increase cerebral blood flow [22, 23]. Together these processes may act like a radiator by removing hyperthermic blood from specific areas while introducing cooler blood from the lungs and extremities, thereby cooling cortical surfaces through convection. It is also hypothesized that the gaping of the mouth and deep inhalation during a yawn cools venous blood draining from the nasal and oral orifices into the cavernous sinus, which surrounds the internal carotid artery supplying blood to the rest of the brain. Thus, the temperature of the air is proposed to give a yawn its utility, not the air's composition.

Empirical Support for the 'Brain Cooling Hypothesis'

Initial support for the brain cooling hypothesis came from a report showing that nasal breathing and direct forehead cooling diminished the incidence of yawning in humans [7]. Given that previous research has shown nasal breathing and forehead cooling each reduce brain temperature [6, 24], it was suggested that the need for yawning may have been eliminated when the brain was sufficiently cooled by nasal cavity airflow or arterial blood supply. Recent research has shown that brain surface temperature can be lowered by mechanical introduction of cool air into the nasal cavity [25], and further evidence using intracranial thermocouples demonstrates nasal inhalation can reduce frontal lobe brain temperature by as much as 0.8°C [24]. Likewise, forehead cooling reduces the temperature of the blood in cutaneous and subcutaneous venous plexuses, and this cooled blood can be transported through venous communications into the venous plexuses of the dura matter [6]. Forehead cooling also enhances dissipation of heat from the skull, and the cooling of venous blood by the skin can in turn alter arterial (carotid) blood supply to the brain.

In order to directly test the brain cooling hypothesis, more recent research has now investigated actual changes in brain and body temperature before and after yawning. In a case report of two women suffering from chronic bouts of yawning, one woman recorded her oral temperature before and after yawning episodes. She reported the onset of a yawning episode occurred during mild hyperthermia (37.5°C), and then resulted in an average decrease in body temperature of roughly 0.4°C following each yawning attack [26]. In addition, both women reported that nasal breathing and forehead cooling (i.e. behavioral brain cooling methods) provided symptom relief and/or postponement of yawning attacks. Thus, empirical evidence reveals that excessive yawning reduces human body temperature. To more explicitly investigate the potential brain cooling effects of yawning, Shoup et al. [27] took continuous measures of brain temperature before and after yawning by implanting rats with thermocoupled temperature probes in the frontal cortex. Consistent with the predictions of the brain cooling hypothesis, spontaneous yawning was triggered in response to rapid increases in brain temperature (+0.12°C), followed by corresponding decreases in temperature immediately following a yawn. These results confirm the hypothesis that yawning produces cerebral cooling. While ±0.12°C might seem trivial, this amounts to roughly 25% of the circadian variance in brain temperature among humans [12].

Further Predictions and Support of the Brain Cooling Model

This evidence suggests the mechanism that triggers yawning lies within a hierarchy of neural structures controlling temperature regulation, offering numerous testable predictions. For one, it is expected that yawning should occur in a narrow range of ambient temperatures (i.e. a thermal window) [7, 8]. Yawns should increase in frequency as ambient temperature approaches body temperature, but should cease when ambient temperatures reach or exceed body temperature because they would no longer result in cooling. It is assumed that during the rise in ambient temperature, the body is heating, stimulating thermoregulatory mechanisms to control temperatures within a normal range. Likewise, when temperatures fall below a certain point, yawning would no longer be beneficial because sending a wave of unusually cool blood to the brain would be maladaptive.

The first prediction was recently tested using budgerigars *(Melopsittacus undulatus)* as an avian model [9]. Results showed that budgerigars' yawning rates were significantly influenced by increasing ambient temperatures, providing the first documented evidence that yawning may be a temperature regulating mechanism in birds. More specifically, yawning frequency increased during rising ambient temperature, but when temperature approached body temperature, yawning began to diminish as other evaporative heat loss behaviors became prevalent. In order to distinguish between whether yawning was triggered due to exposure to higher or increasing ambient temperature, or simply by change in temperature (irrespective of direction), a more recent study manipulated ambient temperature in both directions and confirmed that yawning occurred significantly more during high-increasing temperatures compared to decreasing temperatures [28]. In addition, yawning was positively correlated with ambient temperature and occurred significantly more often in the presence of other thermoregulatory behaviors.

Existing research suggests that excessive yawning is not always indicative of sleep deprivation or sleep disorder, and may be a more important symptom of an individual's inability to properly maintain thermal homeostasis [29]. Gallup and Gallup [8] have reviewed mounting evidence showing that yawning occurs before, during and after instances of heat stress, hyperthermia and abnormal thermoregulation. For instance, drugs that increase brain temperature produce excessive yawning (e.g. certain serotonin reuptake inhibitors), while drugs that produce hypothermia (e.g. opioids) inhibit yawning. Excessive yawning is also symptomatic of conditions that increase brain and/or core body temperature, such as central nervous system damage, epilepsy, migraine headaches, multiple sclerosis, and stress and anxiety. It is hypothesized that frequent yawning is a symptom of an inability to effectively maintain optimal brain thermoregulation, and therefore yawning may be indicative of hyperthermia. Recent research on patients with multiple sclerosis, a documented thermoregulatory disorder, shows that over 1 out of 3 individuals indicate that yawning provides temporary relief of their MS symptoms [30]. Similarly, recent pilot data show that some epileptic patients notice yawning before and after seizures and 50% of these patients reported that yawning made their symptoms slightly better [Gallup AC, Gallup Jr. GG, unpubl. data]. It is proposed that the alleviatory effects described by such patients are a result of cerebral cooling.

Conclusions

Overall, this research provides strong support for the view that yawning stimulates or facilitates cortical arousal, with growing evidence suggesting the biological function of yawning among homeotherms is central thermoregulation. Comparative research from birds, rats and humans shows that yawning reduces brain and body temperature, is influenced by the range and direction of ambient temperature change, and is inhibited by methods of behavioral cooling (e.g. nasal breathing and forehead cooling). Further support comes from the fact that excessive yawning is frequently associated with conditions of heat stress, hyperthermia and abnormal thermoregulation, and drugs and other conditions that promote increases in brain and/or body temperature have been shown to increase yawning frequency. This model is powerful because it not only integrates a great deal of seemingly diverse information about yawning from a variety of species, but it can also be used to generate numerous testable predictions.

The evidence presented in this chapter cannot be overlooked or ignored, as it offers direct application for medical research and diagnosis, as well as providing critical insights to sleep medicine. Yawning has well-documented thermoregulatory consequences, and the use of thermocoupled probes in rats confirms the hypothesis that yawning provides cerebral cooling. The fact of the matter is that the 'brain cooling hypothesis' is no longer a topic of debate.

References

1 Baenninger R: Some comparative aspects of yawning in *Betta splendens*, *Homo sapiens*, *Panthera leo*, and *Papio sphinx*. J Comp Psychol 1987;101:349–354.

2 Provine RR: Yawning as a stereotyped action pattern and releasing stimulus. Ethology 1986;72:109–122.

3 Provine RR: Yawning. Am Sci 2005;93:532–539.

4 Provine RR, Tate BC, Geldmacher LL: Yawning: no effect of 3–5% CO_2, 100% O_2, and exercise. Behav Neural Biol 1987;48:382–393.

5 Baenninger R: On yawning and its functions. Psychonomic Bull Rev 1997;4:198–207.

6 Zenker W, Kubik S: Brain cooling in humans – anatomical considerations. Anat Embryol (Berl) 1996; 193:1–13.

7 Gallup AC, Gallup GG Jr: Yawning as a brain cooling mechanism: nasal breathing and forehead cooling diminish the incidence of contagious yawning. Evol Psychol 2007;5:92–101.

8 Gallup AC, Gallup Jr GG: Yawning and thermoregulation. Physiol Behav 2008;95:10–16.

9 Gallup AC, Miller ML, Clark AB: Yawning and thermoregulation in budgerigars (*Melopsittacus undulatus*). Anim Behav 2009;77:109–113.

10 Provine RR, Hamernik HB, Curchack BB: Yawning: relation to sleeping and stretching in humans. Ethology 1986;76:152–160.

11 Zilli I, Giganti F, Salzarulo P: Yawning in morning and evening types. Physiol Behav 2007;91:218–222.

12 Landolt HP, Moser S, Wiesen HG, Borbeley AA, Dijk DJ: Intracranial temperature across 24 hour sleep wake cycles in humans. Neuroreport 1995; 6:913–917.

13 Everson CA, Smith CB, Sokoloff L: Effects of prolonged sleep deprivation on local rates of cerebral energy metabolism in freely moving rats. J Neurosci 1994;14:6769–6778.

14 Krauchi K, Cajochen C, Wirz-Justice A: A relationship between heat loss and sleepiness: effects of postural change and melatonin administration. J Appl Physiol 1997;83:134–139.

15 Krauchi K, Cajochen C, Wirz-Justice A: Thermophysiological aspects of the three-process-model of sleepiness regulation. Clin J Sport Med 2005;24:287–300.

16 Krauchi K, Vollenweider S, Muller S, Renz C, Schachinger H, Wirz-Justice A: Thermoregulatory dissociation of awareness and psychomotor vigilance (abstract). Sleep 2006;29(suppl):A34.

17 Argiolas A, Melis MR: The neuropharmacology of yawning. Eur J Pharmacol 1998;343:1–16.

18 Cooper KE: Molecular biology of thermoregulation: some historical perspectives on thermoregulation. J Appl Physiol 2002;92:1717–1724.

19 Greco M, Baenninger R: Effects of yawning and related activities on skin conductance and heart rate. Physiol Behav 1991;50:1067–1069.

20 Guggisberg AG, Mathis J, Herrmann US, Hess CW: The functional relationship between yawning and vigilance. Behav Brain Res 2007;179:159–166.

21 Askenasy JJM, Askenasy N: Inhibition of muscle sympathetic nerve activity during yawning. Clin Auton Res 1996;6:237–239.

22 Askenasy JJM: Is yawning an arousal defense reflex? J Psychol 1989;123:609–621.

23 Zajonc RB: Emotion and facial efference: a theory reclaimed. Science 1985;288:15–21.

24 Mariak Z, White MD, Lewko J, Lyson T, Piekarski P: Direct cooling of the human brain by heat loss from the upper respiratory tract. J Appl Physiol 1999;87: 1609–1613.

25 Harris BA, Andrews PJD, Murray GD: Enhanced upper respiratory tract airflow and head fanning reduce brain temperature in brain-injured, mechanically ventilated patients: a randomized, crossover, factorial trial. Br J Anesth 2007;98:93–99.

26 Gallup GG Jr, Gallup AC: Yawning and thermoregulation: two case histories of chronic, debilitating yawning. Sleep Breath, E-pub ahead of print.

27 Shoup ML, Gallup AC, Gallup GG Jr, McNay EC: Yawning cools the brain. Under review.

28 Gallup AC, Miller ML, Clark AB: The direction and range of ambient temperature influences yawning in budgerigars (*Melopsittacus undulatus*). J Comp Psychol, in press.

29 Gallup AC: Misconceptions regarding excessive yawning and sleep deprivation; in Fulke P, Vaughan S (eds): Sleep Deprivation: Causes, Effects, and Treatment. Hauppauge, Nova Science, in press.

30 Gallup AC, Gallup GG Jr, Feo C: Yawning, sleep, and symptom relief in patients with multiple sclerosis. Sleep Med, in press.

A.C. Gallup
Department of Biological Sciences, Binghamton University
Binghamton, NY–13902 USA
Tel. +1 518 727 2473, Fax +1 607 777 6521
E-Mail a.c.gallup@gmail.com

Walusinski O (ed): The Mystery of Yawning in Physiology and Disease.
Front Neurol Neurosci. Basel, Karger, 2010, vol 28, pp 90–106

Neurophamacology of Yawning

Gregory T. Collins[a] · Jose R. Eguibar[b]

[a]Department of Pharmacology, University of Michigan, Ann Arbor, Mich., USA; [b]Instituto de Fisiología, Benemérita Universidad Autónoma de Puebla, Puebla, México

Abstract

Yawning is a common behavioral event that is observed in humans, as well as other mammals, birds and reptiles. In humans, yawning often occurs just before bed and upon waking up, and is also associated with tedious or boring situations. Although the physiologic roles of yawning have yet to be fully elucidated, the past 50 years of research has led to a much greater understanding of the neuropharmacologic regulation of yawning. While many of the early studies concluded that yawning was primarily driven by changes in cholinergic neurotransmission, we now know that numerous neurotransmitters and neurohormones are involved in the mediation of yawning, including acetylcholine, dopamine, glutamate, serotonin, oxytocin, GABA, opioids, adrenergics, nitric oxide, as well as the proopiomelanocortin-derived peptides ACTH and α-MSH. Furthermore, antagonist interaction studies have clearly defined at least 3 distinct neural pathways involved in the induction of yawning, as well as the hierarchical order through which these different neurotransmitter systems interact to regulate yawning. The following sections will discuss the state of knowledge for each of the major neurotransmitters and neurohormones involved in the regulation of yawning, their interactions with one another, and their place in the hierarchical organization of yawning.

Yawning is a phylogenetically conserved behavior, observed in mammals, birds and reptiles; it is essentially defined as a paroxysm of the respiratory cycle characterized by a standard cascade of movements over a 5- to 10-second period [1], with 3 distinct phases. Yawning is initiated by a wide opening of the mouth with an ample, slow and deep inspiration, followed by a brief interruption of ventilation fluxes once the thorax is full (the so-called acme state, which is often is accompanied by limb stretching and eye occlusion) and concluding with a short expiration, accompanied by the relaxation of all participating muscles. In the case of humans, yawning is also accompanied by a great expansion of the pharynx and larynx, and a maximal abduction of the vocal cords, with inspiration occurring essentially through the mouth. Although the duration of a yawn in a given individual appears to be fixed, it can be modulated voluntarily. Furthermore, it is important to note that yawning is also accompanied by an opening of the eustachian tubes, a brief lowering of hearing acuity, as well as the opening of the stomach cardia resulting in an influx of intragastric air that is responsible for the sensation of abdominal fullness occasionally associated with yawning. Thus, yawning should not be thought of simply as the opening one's mouth, but rather a generalized stretching of muscles, particularly those of the respiratory tract, such as the diaphragm, intercostals, and those of the face and neck [2].

Although yawning is often associated with tedious or boring situations such as reading, traveling on public transport, driving, waiting or watching monotonous videos [3–5], yawning should not be thought of as simply a sign of boredom. For instance, yawning is thought to act as an alarm signal to warn drivers about the risk of falling asleep while driving a vehicle, particularly on long straight highways [6–9], suggesting that yawning may play a role in affecting arousal states. In fact, in humans yawning occurs most frequently during the transition from one state of arousal to another, such as just before bedtime and immediately after waking up, with the later particularly associated with stretching of the forelimbs and trunk [4, 10, 11]. Interestingly, in anesthetized rats, instances of inspiration and mouth opening (i.e. yawning) were preceded by cortical arousal, further supporting the notion that yawning is associated with changes in arousal states [12].

In a series of studies, Anías et al. [13] have clearly demonstrated the influence of circadian rhythms on the frequency of yawning, as the peak incidence of yawning in an inbred high-yawning subline of rats occurred just before the dark phase, regardless of the light-dark schedule. The peak in yawning disappeared when rats were subjected to constant light conditions, suggesting that this pattern of yawning is not endogenously generated. Interestingly, when these rats were further subjected to a restricted feeding schedule of just 2 h per day, a significant increase in yawning was observed just prior to feeding, suggesting that the anticipation of food is capable of functioning as a zeitgeber for the circadian regulation of yawning [14]. Similar instances of anticipatory yawning have been reported just before feeding in zoo animals, such as carnivores, fish and monkeys, as well as in wild hyenas, which yawn repeatedly while circling a dead animal just before eating it [15, 16]. These peaks in yawning are correlated with increased corticoid levels.

In addition, yawning has recently been hypothesized to play a role in thermoregulation dysfunctions, insofar as increases in yawning are observed when brain and/or core body temperatures are elevated, and decreases in yawning are observed as temperatures return to normal, suggesting that yawning may provide a compensatory cooling mechanism [17]. Similar effects are seen with D_2-like agonists which increase yawning over low doses, and induce hypothermia at higher doses that also corresponded to decreases in yawning [18]. Although a causal relation was not implied, these findings provide further support for the notion that there is an association between the regulation of core body temperature and the frequency of yawning.

Finally, it is well know that yawning is contagious in humans. Provine [19] has reported that 55% of spectators viewing a brief video of 30 successive yawns yawned themselves within a period of a few seconds to 5 min. Additionally, it appears that observing the complete face of the yawner is necessary to induce yawning, as viewing only part of the face, such as a wide-open mouth, failed to trigger replication. Thus, Provine et al. [19, 20] concluded that contagious yawning in humans depends on a multimodal perception of the entire facial configuration, combined with audible respiratory movements and the coordinating dynamics. Studies in macaque monkeys have linked this ability to imitate behaviors to a group of neurons within the ventral premotor cortex, called mirror neurons, whose activity is correlated not only with the performance of specific behaviors, but also the observation of these behaviors in other individuals, suggesting that mirror neurons may provide the neurophysiologic foundation for contagious yawning in monkeys as well as humans [21].

Clearly, yawning is not a simple behavior, but rather a common response to a variety of environmental and physiologic stimuli, many of which will be described in greater detail in other chapters of this book. This chapter will instead focus on what is known about the neuropharmacologic regulation of yawning, as well as the hierarchical organization and interactions of the major neurotransmitter systems involved in the induction and regulation of yawning (fig. 1; table 1).

Major Neurotransmitters Involved in the Induction of Yawning

Adrenocorticotropic Hormone and α-Melanocyte-Stimulating Hormone

One of the earliest accounts of pharmacologically-induced yawning was provided by Ferrari et al. [22], who described a series of behavioral effects characterized by increases in stretching, yawning and grooming that occurred following the intracisternal administration of either adrenocorticotropic hormone (ACTH) or α-melanocyte-stimulating hormone (α-MSH): two of the centrally active peptide hormones that are formed by the processing of proopiomelanocortin (POMC) in the brain and pituitary. Although the fact that yawning is abolished by hypophysectomy suggests that an intact pituitary gland is necessary for ACTH to induce yawning [23], other studies have suggested that the hypothalamus is the primary site of action as increases in yawning are observed following the microinjection of ACTH into several hypothalamic nuclei [24], including the paraventricular nucleus (PVN), dorsomedial nucleus, ventromedial nucleus and anterior hypothalamus [25]. Dose-dependent decreases in yawning induced by the intra-PVN administration of ACTH are observed following microinjection of the melanocortin-4 receptor antagonist, HS014, into the PVN suggesting that activation of melanocortin-4 receptors within the PVN is sufficient for ACTH to induce yawning [25]. However, as yawning induced by the intracerebroventricular (ICV) administration of ACTH is not affected by the electrolytic lesion of the PVN [26], it is likely that multiple hypothalamic nuclei are involved in the mediation of ACTH- and α-MSH-induced yawning.

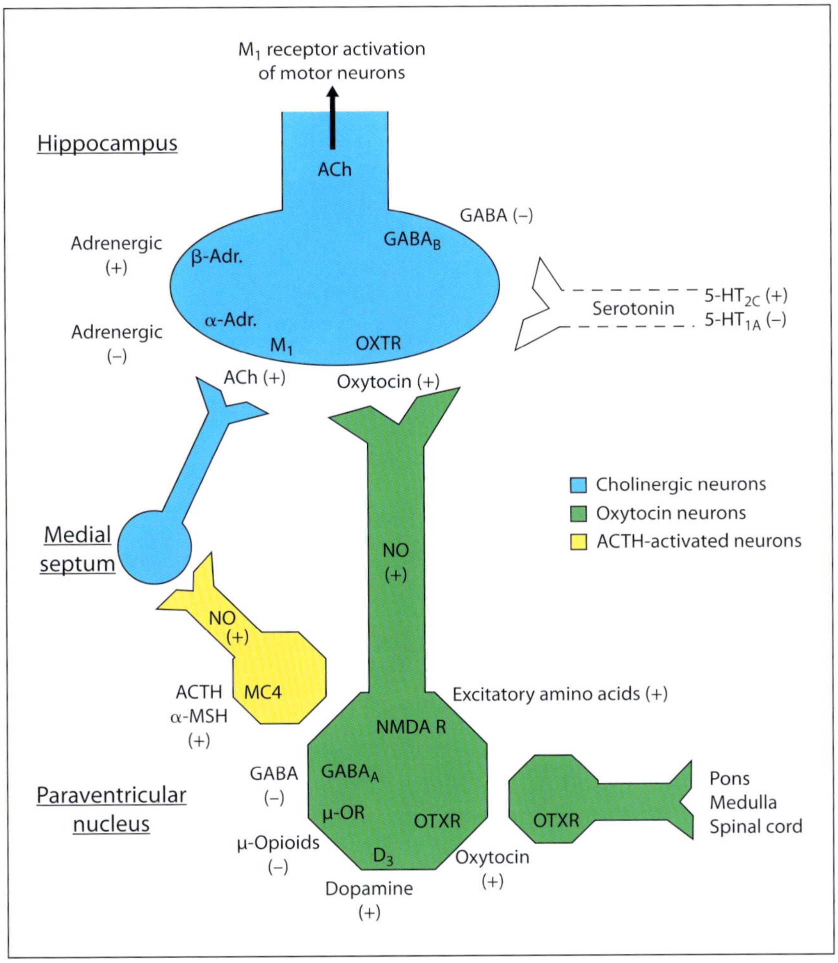

Fig. 1. Schematic representation of the neurotransmitters and receptor subtypes involved in the mediation of yawning. The main neural pathways that have been hypothesized to be involved in the regulation of yawning include: (1) two separate groups of oxytocinergic neurons projecting from the PVN to the CA1 region of the hippocampus, or the pons, medulla or spinal cord; (2) ACTH-/α-MSH-activated neurons projecting from the PVN to the hippocampus via activation of septo-hippocampal cholinergic neurons; (3) direct activation of septo-hippocampal/hippocampal cholinergic neurons; (4) a serotonergic-cholinergic pathway that has yet to be identified. Neurotransmitter systems/receptors that are capable of inducing or enhancing yawning are denoted by a (+), whereas those that are involved in the inhibition of yawning are denoted by a (–). See text for details regarding the interactions of these neurotransmitter systems.

Despite the fact that the hypothalamus, and in particular the PVN, is known to be involved in the induction of yawning by a variety of pharmacologic stimuli, including dopamine and oxytocin (see later sections), it is important to note that ACTH-induced yawning is not affected by dopamine D_2-like or oxytocin receptor antagonists [27, 28]. Although these findings suggest that the neurons involved

Table 1. Neurotransmitters involved in the regulation of yawning

Neurotransmitter	Effect of yawning	Receptor(s)	Brain region
ACTH/MSH	stimulatory	MC_4	hypothalamus
Acetylcholine	stimulatory	M_1	HI
Oxytocin	stimulatory	OXTR	PVN, HI
Nitric oxide	stimulatory	n.a.	PVN, others
Dopamine	stimulatory inhibitory	D_3 D_2	PVN
Excitatory AA	stimulatory	NMDA	PVN
Serotonin	stimulatory inhibitory	$5\text{-}HT_{2C}$ $5\text{-}HT_2/5\text{-}HT_{1A}$	n.d. n.d.
Opioid	inhibitory	μ-opioid	PVN, others
GABA	inhibitory	$GABA_A/GABA_B$	PVN, HI
Adrenergic	enhancing inhibitory	α_2-adrenergic β-adrenergic	n.d. n.d.

HI = Hippocampus; PVN = paraventricular nucleus of the hypothalamus; AA = amino acids.

in the mediation of ACTH-induced yawning are independent of those that mediate dopaminergic and oxytocinergic yawning, the induction of yawning by ACTH and α-MSH does not occur via completely autonomous mechanisms. For instance, similar to yawning induced by oxytocin, or D_2-like agonists, yawning induced by ACTH and α-MSH is inhibited by centrally active anticholinergics, such as atropine [22]. In total, these findings suggest that ACTH- and α-MSH-induced yawning results from the activation of melanocortin-4 receptors within a variety of hypothalamic nuclei, and although these receptors appear to be located on neurons that are distinct from those that involved in other forms or yawning (i.e. dopaminergic or oxytocinergic), ACTH-induced yawning appears to be mediated by a downstream activation of cholinergic neurotransmission that may be common for all forms of yawning.

Acetylcholine

A role for cholinergic neurons in the mediation of yawning was first suggested after dose-dependent increases in yawning were observed following systemic administration of the acetylcholinesterase inhibitor, physostigmine, and the direct muscarinic receptor agonist, pilocarpine [29], effects that have been replicated with a variety of centrally active, but not peripheral acetylcholinesterase inhibitors [30–32]. Further support for a role of central muscarinic receptors in the induction of yawning was provided by antagonist interaction studies in which dose-dependent decreases in physostigmine-induced yawning were observed following administration of the centrally active cholinergic muscarinic receptor antagonist, scopolamine, but not the peripherally active muscarinic receptor antagonist methylscopolamine or the nicotinic receptor antagonist mecamylamine [29, 33, 34]. A specific role for the muscarinic M_1 receptor subtype in the induction of yawning was later proposed based on the findings that M_1 receptor agonists, such as RS-86 and YM796, induced dose-depended increases in yawning, whereas moderately selective M_1 antagonists, such as pirenzepine, inhibited yawning induced by either physostigmine or direct M_1 agonists [35–37].

In addition to supporting a role for M_1 cholinergic receptors in the induction of yawning, antagonist interaction studies have also provided evidence suggesting that septo-hippocampal cholinergic neurons play an important role in the mediation of yawning induced by a variety of pharmacologic agents. For instance, not only does ACTH- and α-MSH-induced yawning correspond to an enhancement of hippocampal acetylcholine turnover rates, but these ACTH- and α-MSH-induced increases in yawning are also blocked by centrally active cholinergic antagonists, such as scopolamine and atropine [22, 36, 38]. In addition, muscarinic antagonists have also been shown to inhibit yawning induced by oxytocin, dopamine D_2-like agonists, such as apomorphine, and 5-HT_2 receptor agonists, such as trifluoromethylphenylpiperazine (TFMPP) [33, 34, 36, 39, 40]. When taken together with the fact that decreases in apomorphine-induced yawning are observed after medial-septal lesions which interrupt the septo-hippocampal pathway [41], these findings point to a central role of septo-hippocampal cholinergic neurons as a site of action for the induction of cholinergic yawning, as well as a common downstream mediator of yawning induced by a variety of pharmacologic mechanisms.

Oxytocin

The first evidence in support of a direct role for oxytocin receptors in the induction of yawning was provided by microinjection studies in which dose-dependent increases in yawning were observed following microinjection of oxytocin into the PVN, as well as the CA1 region of the hippocampus [42], effects that were blocked by the ICV or intra-PVN administration of oxytocin receptor antagonists, such as d(CH2)5Tyr(Me)-[Orn8]vasotocin [26, 27, 36, 43, 44], as well as the systemic administration of anticholinergics [36, 39]. In addition to their capacity to inhibit oxytocin-induced yawning, oxytocin antagonists have also been shown to inhibit yawning induced by dopamine D_2-like agonists, such as apomorphine and N-methyl-D-aspartic acid (NMDA); however, these effects are only observed following ICV and not intra-PVN administration [44], suggesting that these effects are mediated by blockade of oxytocin receptors outside of the PVN. In addition, although electrolytic lesion of the PVN is capable of inhibiting the induction of yawning by the ICV administration of either oxytocin or apomorphine [26], medial-septal lesions inhibited apomorphine-induced yawning (intra-PVN or ICV), but failed to affect yawning induced by either intra-PVN or ICV oxytocin [41]. When taken together with the finding that the induction of yawning by D_2-like agonists, such as apomorphine, also corresponds to increases in hippocampal oxytocin [26, 27, 45], these findings suggest that oxytocin neurons originating in the PVN and projecting to the hippocampus play an integral role in the mediation of yawning induced by D_2-like agonists and NMDA, the details of which will be described in later sections. However, the fact that medial-septal lesions failed to inhibit oxytocin-induced yawning suggests that a functional septo-hippocampal pathway is not necessary for oxytocin to induce yawning, raising the possibility that oxytocinergic neurons projecting from the PVN to structures such as the pons, medulla oblongata or spinal cord may also be capable of inducing yawning when stimulated by oxytocin [41 and references therein].

Nitric Oxide

In addition to their work demonstrating the importance of oxytocin in the mediation of yawning, Drs. Melis and Argiolas have also provided clear evidence of a central role of nitric oxide (NO) in the mediation of yawning [for review, see: 46]. Early evidence suggested that NO-induced yawning resulted from increased oxytocinergic neurotransmission, as yawning induced by the intra-PVN administration of NO donors, such as sodium nitroprusside, hydroxylamine and nitroglycerin, was blocked by the ICV administration of oxytocin antagonists [47, 48]. Further support for a role of NO in the mediation of yawning was provided by studies in which the intra-PVN administration of NO synthase inhibitors, such as NG-nitro-L-arginine methyl ester (L-NAME), were shown to be capable of inhibiting yawning induced by either apomorphine or oxytocin [49, 50], suggesting that in addition to stimulating yawning, NO signaling also plays an important role in the mediation of yawning induced by a variety of other mechanisms. This notion was later confirmed by studies in which a clear correspondence between the induction of yawning (by apomorphine, oxytocin and NMDA) and increased levels of NO_2 (a reliable indicator of NO production) within the PVN was demonstrated [51, 52]. However, it is important to note that while the intra-PVN administration of L-NAME blocks yawning that is mediated by activation of oxytocinergic neurons within the PVN (i.e. D_2-like agonist-, NMDA- and oxytocin-induced yawning), the ICV administration of L-NAME has also been shown to block yawning that is not mediated by PVN oxytocinergic neurons (i.e. ACTH- and $5\text{-}HT_{2C}$ agonist-induced yawning [53, 54]). Together, these studies suggest that increases in NO signaling likely play a more general role in the mediation of yawning induced by a variety of mechanisms, the details of which will be described in later sections.

Dopamine

Although a variety of neurotransmitter systems are known to be involved in the regulation of yawning, perhaps none has received as much attention as the capacity of dopaminergic drugs to induce yawning. Since it was initially described by Mogilnicka and Klimek [55], hundreds of studies have investigated the phenomenon of D_2-like agonist-induced yawning, with many of the early studies focusing on the interactions of dopaminergic and cholinergic systems in the induction of yawning. For instance, in addition to being inhibited by centrally active D_2-like antagonists, such as spiroperidol, haloperidol and sulpiride, D_2-like agonist-induced yawning is also blocked by centrally active anticholinergics, such as scopolamine. Moreover, when combined with the inability of D_2-like antagonists to inhibit physostigmine-induced yawning, these studies support the notion that dopaminergic yawning is mediated by a downstream increase in cholinergic activity [56–58], similar to what has been described for ACTH- and oxytocin- induced yawning. Although early microinjection studies suggested that the induction of yawning by D_2-like agonists may be mediated by their actions in the striatum or septum [59, 60], subsequent studies demonstrated that apomorphine was capable of inducing yawning when injected into the PVN at doses approximately 5–40 times lower than those that were required to induce yawning in the striatum or septum [61], suggesting that the PVN may play a central role in the mediation of dopaminergic yawning, as had been previously described for oxytocin [42].

Subsequent studies by Drs. Argiolas and Melis provided several lines of evidence that clearly demonstrate the involvement of PVN oxytocinergic neurons in the mediation of D_2-like agonist-induced yawning. For instance, in addition to increasing yawning, apomorphine has also been shown to increase hippocampal oxytocin levels, two effects that are similarly inhibited by D_2-like antagonists [45]. Moreover, although apomorphine-induced yawning is prevented by electrolytic lesion of the PVN or the ICV administration of the oxytocin antagonists [26, 43], D_2-like antagonists fail to alter oxytocin-induced yawning [27, 42], suggesting that oxytocin plays an important role in the downstream mediation of dopaminergic yawning. Similarly, the induction of yawning by apomorphine also corresponds to increased NO_2 levels within the PVN, an effect that is blocked by D_2-like antagonists and NO synthase inhibitors, but not oxytocin antagonists, which only block yawning [52]. Collectively, these studies suggest that dopaminergic yawning is induced via activation of D_2-like receptors within the PVN, resulting in NO- and oxytocin-dependent increases in hippocampal cholinergic activity.

In addition to studies aimed at elucidating the neurotransmitters and pathways involved in the mediation of D_2-like agonist-induced yawning, a significant effort has been put forth to identify the receptor(s) responsible for the induction and subsequent inhibition of yawning by D_2-like agonists. Early hypotheses attributed the induction of yawning to increased cholinergic activity resulting from the activation of pre-synaptic D_2 receptors, whereas the subsequent inhibition of yawning was thought to be mediated by post-synaptic D_2 receptors or the concomitant activation of D_1 receptors [34, 62, 63]. However, based on the inability of pharmacologic manipulations that alter synaptic dopamine levels to affect D_2-like agonist-induced yawning, as well as the finding that apomorphine-induced yawning did not correspond to changes in synaptic dopamine levels, Stahle and Ungerstedt proposed that the biphasic nature of D_2-like agonist-induced yawning was mediated by multiple post-synaptic D_2 receptors with differing sensitivities, and not pre-synaptic D_2 receptors [34, 62–68].

Subsequent to this change in thinking, a number of studies reported dose-dependent increases in yawning following administration of a wide variety of D_3-preferring agonists, such as pramipexole, PD-128,907, 7-OH-DPAT, quinpirole and quinelorane, but not the D_2-preferring agonist sumanirole [18, 40, 69], raising the possibility that the D_3 receptor was involved in the mediation of yawning. Specific roles for the D_3 and D_2 receptors in the mediation of yawning were later confirmed by a series of antagonist studies in which D_3-selective antagonists, such as PG01037 and SB-277011A, were shown to selectively inhibit the induction of yawning; the D_2-preferring antagonist L-741,626 was shown to selectively reverse of the inhibition of yawning; and mixed D_2/D_3 antagonists, such as haloperidol and raclopride, were shown to produce rightward shifts in both the ascending and descending limbs of the dose-response curves for D_3-preferring agonist-induced yawning [40, 69–72]. Thus, while dopaminergic yawning involves downstream increases in oxytocin, NO and acetylcholine signaling, these findings strongly suggest that the induction of yawning is mediated by the selective activation of D_3 receptors, whereas the inhibition of yawning observed with higher doses of D_2-like agonists is mediated by the concomitant activation of D_2 receptors.

Excitatory Amino Acids

As mentioned in previous sections, excitatory amino acids (such as NMDA) are also capable of inducing yawning, an effect that was first described following the intra-PVN administration of NMDA for the purpose of studying grooming behavior [73]. Although it was unclear at the time, these increases in yawning were later shown to be NMDA-specific, as yawning was observed following the intra-PVN administration of NMDA, but not α-amino-3-hydroxyl-5-methyl-4-isoxazole-propionate (AMPA) or (±)-1-aminocyclopentane-trans-1,3-dicarboxylic acid (ACPD) agonists of the AMPA and metabotropic glutamate receptors, respectively [44]. Furthermore, in addition to being blocked by variety of NMDA receptor antagonists, including MK-801 [44, 74], NMDA-induced yawning has also been shown to be dose-dependently inhibited by the ICV, but not intra-PVN, administration of oxytocin antagonists, as well as the

ICV or intra-PVN administration of L-NAME [44, 75, 76], suggesting that NMDA-induced yawning is mediated by the activation of oxytocinergic neurons within the PVN in a NO-dependent manner. Importantly though, NMDA-induced yawning is not blocked by D_2-like antagonists, just as apomorphine-induced yawning is not blocked by NMDA antagonists [74, 76]. Thus, although NMDA- and D_2-like agonist-induced yawning appear to be similarly mediated by the activation of oxytocinergic neurons with in the PVN, in an NO-dependent manner, the influences of NMDA and dopamine on yawning appear to be independent of each other. Moreover, these findings provide further evidence for a central role of oxytocinergic neurons within the PVN insofar as they are responsible for the integration of inputs from a variety of neurotransmitter systems that are involved in the mediation of yawning.

Serotonin

Serotonin (5-HT) was first proposed to be involved in the regulation of yawning by Urba-Holmgren et al. [77], who described an enhancement of physostigmine-induced yawning following treatment with the selective 5-HT reuptake inhibitor citalopram, an effect that was blocked by the 5-HT receptor antagonist, metergoline. Although the mechanism by which 5-HT affected yawning was unclear at the time, more recent studies have suggested that 5-HT may play multiple roles in the mediation of yawning. For example, dose-dependent increases in yawning are observed following the systemic, but not intra-PVN, administration of 5-HT_{2C}-preferring agonists, such as m-CPP, TFMPP and MK 212, effects that are blocked by 5-HT_2 receptor antagonists, such as mianserin and ritanserin [40, 53, 78, 79]. However, unlike with D_2-like agonist- and NMDA-induced yawning, 5-HT_{2C} agonist-induced yawning is not reduced by D_2-like antagonists, oxytocin antagonists or the intra-PVN administration of NO synthase inhibitors [40, 53, 79], suggesting that serotonergic yawning is mediated by the activation of 5-HT_{2C} receptors located outside the PVN, rather than an interaction with oxytocinergic neurons within the PVN. However, it is interesting to note that despite these important differences, reductions in m-CPP- and TFMPP-induced yawning are observed following the ICV administration of NO synthase inhibitors [53], suggesting that serotonergic yawning is mediated by increases in NO signaling, although not within the PVN. In addition, m-CPP- and TFMPP-induced yawning appears to be mediated by the downstream activation of cholinergic systems as yawning is inhibited by the systemic administration of anticholinergics, such as scopolamine [40, 80]. Although it is unclear if serotonergic yawning is mediated by septo-hippocampal cholinergic neurons, these findings provide further support for a integral role for cholinergic neurotransmission in the coordination of yawning induced by a variety of neurotransmitter systems.

In addition to its role in the stimulation of yawning, several lines of evidence have suggested that 5-HT may also have a more general role in the tonic inhibition of yawning. For instance, although depletion of endogenous 5-HT by p-chlorophenylalanine or the selective lesioning of serotonergic neurons by 5,7-dihydroxytryptamine has been shown to result in an enhancement of D_2-like agonist- and physostigmine-induced yawning, enhancing serotonergic activity through treatment with the 5-HT precursor 5-hydroxytryptophan has been shown to inhibit D_2-like agonist- and physostigmine-induced yawning [81, 82]. Similar inhibitions of dopaminergic, serotonergic and cholinergic yawning have also been observed with 5-HT_{1A} receptor agonists, such as 8-OH-DPAT, S 14506, and S 20499 [80, 83]. Thus, although activation of 5-HT_{2C} receptors results in the induction of yawning through a mechanism unrelated to oxytocin neurotransmission in the PVN, 5-HT_{1A} receptors appear to mediate the general inhibitory effect of 5-HT on yawning induced by a variety of mechanisms.

Major Neurotransmitters Involved in the Modulation of Yawning

Opioids

As discussed previously, the POMC-derived peptides ACTH and α-MSH were some of the first compounds to be shown to induce yawning in laboratory animals [22]; however, it is worth noting that β-endorphin, a POMC derived peptide with μ-opioid agonist activity, has been shown to inhibit ACTH-induced yawning [84, 85], suggesting an inhibitory role for the μ-opioid receptor on yawning. This notion is further supported by a number of studies that have demonstrated the capacity of morphine, a non-peptidic μ-opioid agonist, to inhibit yawning induced by a variety of mechanisms, including ACTH, physostigmine, D_2-like agonists, NMDA and oxytocin, effects that are reversed by the μ-opioid receptor antagonist naloxone [86–90]. Interestingly, although microinjection studies suggest that the inhibitory effects of morphine result from the activation of μ-opioid receptors on oxytocinergic neurons within the PVN [87, 88], the fact that systemically administered morphine is also capable of inhibiting yawning that is not mediated by oxytocin neurotransmission (i.e. ACTH and physostigmine) [22, 89] suggests that μ-opioid receptors in other brain regions may also be involved in the tonic inhibition of yawning. In addition, it is interesting to note that increases in yawning have been used for the identification and characterization of morphine withdrawal in humans and laboratory animals dating back to the 1930s [91–93].

GABA

Although it has not been extensively studied, a handful of studies have suggested that γ-amminobutyric acid (GABA) is also involved in the regulation of yawning. Curiously, although the γ-amminobutyric acid transaminase inhibitor, γ-acetylenic-GABA, has been shown to increase spontaneous yawning, studies of the effects of $GABA_A$ and $GABA_B$ agonists on yawning have generally suggested that GABAergic receptors have an inhibitory rather than stimulatory influence on yawning [94]. For example, systemic administration of $GABA_A$ agonists, such as muscimol, or the $GABA_B$ agonists, such as baclofen, have been shown to inhibit physostigmine-induced yawning, effects that are reversed by the $GABA_A$ antagonist bicuculline and the $GABA_B$ antagonist phaclofen, respectively [94, 95]. Despite the similarities in these effects, however, several lines of evidence suggest that $GABA_A$ and $GABA_B$ receptors may be exerting their inhibitory effects at different stages of the pathway(s) responsible for the induction of yawning. For instance, although the intra-PVN administration of the $GABA_A$ agonist muscimol inhibits apomorphine-, NMDA- and oxytocin-induced yawning in a NO-dependent and bicuculline-sensitive manner, baclofen fails to affect apomorphine-, NMDA- or oxytocin-induced yawning when administered into the PVN [51, 96]. Thus, although $GABA_A$ receptors located on oxytocinergic neurons in the PVN may be capable of inhibiting yawning, it also appears as though $GABA_B$ receptors located outside of the PVN are capable of inhibiting yawning, possibly through a $GABA_B$ receptor-mediated inhibition of hippocampal acetylcholine activity [97].

Adrenergic

Similar to the capacity of drugs that act on GABA and μ-opioid receptors to affect yawning without inducing it, a variety of adrenergic drugs have been shown to modify yawning induced by other mechanisms. Despite their inability to induce yawning, centrally active β-adrenergic antagonists have generally been shown to enhance yawning, whereas α_2-adrenergic antagonists generally inhibit yawning induced by D_2-like agonists, oxytocin, cholinomimetics, M_1 agonists as well as α-MSH [36, 37, 63, 98, 99]. Curiously, and somewhat less convincingly, α-adrenergic agonists have been reported to inhibit yawning, and β-adrenergic agonists to enhance yawning induced by D_2-like agonists and cholinomimetics [99–101]. Despite these peculiarities, the fact that these adrenergic antagonists are capable of modifying yawning induced by a variety of pathways (i.e. ACTH/α-MSH, PVN oxytocinergic stimulation, and direct cholinergic activation), suggests that the effects of β- and α_2-adrenergic antagonists on yawning likely results from an interaction of adrenergic systems with the septo-hippocampal cholinergic neurons that has been shown to be involved in the coordination and mediation of yawning induced by a variety of neurotransmitter systems.

Conclusions

Although the phenomenon of yawning has fascinated man throughout time, most of the significant advances towards our understanding of the neuropharmacologic regulation of yawning have been made during the past 50 years. We now know that a variety of neurotransmitters and neurohormones are involved in the induction and regulation of yawning, including acetylcholine, dopamine, glutamate, serotonin, oxytocin, GABA, opioids, adrenergics, nitric oxide, as well as the POMC-derived peptides ACTH and α-MSH. Despite this diverse set of neurotransmitters, the majority of yawning is mediated by at least 3 distinct pathways, all of which appear to converge on cholinergic neurons within the hippocampus. In addition, the elegant work of Drs. Argiolas and Melis has demonstrated the importance of the hypothalamus in the regulation of yawning, as many of these neurotransmitters appear to affect yawning through their interactions with oxytocinergic neurons within the PVN. For instance, activation of these oxytocinergic neurons by dopamine, glutamate, nitric oxide and oxytocin is known to induce yawning, whereas inhibition of these neurons by μ-opioids and GABA has been shown to reduce the frequency of yawning. It is important to note that although the effects of ACTH and α-MSH are also mediated by the hypothalamus, the induction of yawning by these peptides does not involve oxytocinergic neurons. Similarly, the induction of yawning by serotonin is also known to occur independently of oxytocinergic neurons within the PVN; however, the brain region(s) responsible for serotonergic yawning are currently unknown. Despite the great advances that have made towards our understanding of the neuropharmacologic regulation of yawning, further studies are needed to fully elucidate how these neurotransmitter systems interact with each other, as well as the specific receptor subtypes and brain regions involved in the induction and inhibition of yawning. Such an understanding would not only advance the use of yawning as a tool for the pharmacologic characterization of receptor subtype-selective agonists, partial-agonists and antagonists, but also further our understanding of how a variety of environmental and pharmacologic manipulations (i.e. dietary conditions or chronic drug treatments) affect the receptor systems involved in the mediation of yawning [71, 102–104]. In addition, a more complete understanding of the neuropharmacologic regulation of yawning could also provide insight into the specific roles of different neurotransmitter systems and/or receptor subtypes in the occurrence of yawning under a variety of physiologic conditions and disease states in which changes in the frequency of yawning are known to occur.

References

1 Barbizet J: Yawning. J Neurol Neurosurg Psychiatry 1958;21:203–209.
2 Baenninger R: On yawning and its functions. Psychonomic Bull Rev 1997;4:198–207.
3 Baenninger R, Greco M: Some antecedents and consequences of yawning. Psychological Record 1991;41:453–460.
4 Greco M, Baenninger R: Effects of yawning and related activities on skin conductance and heart rate. Physiol Behav 1991;50:1067–1069.
5 Provine RR, Hamernik HB: Yawning, Effects of stimulus interest. B Psychonomic Soc 1986;24:437–438.

6 Cummings P, et al: Drowsiness, counter-measures to drowsiness, and the risk of a motor vehicle crash. Inj Prev 2001;7:194–199.
7 Kishida K: Temporal change of subsidiary behavior in monotonous work. J Hum Ergol (Tokyo) 1973;2: 75–89.
8 Koch SW, Koe BK, Bacopoulos NG: Differential effects of the enantiomers of 3-(3-hydroxyphenyl)-N-n-propylpiperidine (3-PPP) at dopamine receptor sites. Eur J Pharmacol 1983;92:279–283.
9 Sakai K, Takahashi Y: Driving and subsidiary behavior of taxi drivers working alternate-day shifts. J Hum Ergol (Tokyo) 1975;4:115–127.
10 Baenninger R, Binkley S, Baenninger M: Field observations of yawning and activity in humans. Physiol Behav 1996;59:421–425.
11 Provine RR, Bamernik HB, Curchack BC: Yawning: Relation to Sleeping and Stretching in Humans. Ethology 1987;76:152–160.
12 Sato-Suzuki I, et al: Cortical arousal induced by microinjection of orexins into the paraventricular nucleus of the rat. Behav Brain Res 2002;128:169–177.
13 Anías J, et al: Circadian variation of yawning behavior. Acta Neurobiol Exp (Wars) 1984;44:179–186.
14 Holmgren B, et al: Food anticipatory yawning rhythm in the rat. Acta Neurobiol Exp (Wars) 1991; 51:97–105.
15 Anderson JR, Wunderlich D: Food-reinforced yawning in Macaca tonkeana. Am J Primatol 1988; 16:165–169.
16 Baenninger R: Some comparative aspects of yawning in Beta splendens, Homo sapiens, Panthera leo, and Papio shinx. J Comp Psychol 1987;101:349–354.
17 Gallup AC, Gallup GG Jr: Yawning and thermoregulation. Physiol Behav 2008;95:10–16.
18 Collins GT, et al: Yawning and hypothermia in rats: effects of dopamine D3 and D2 agonists and antagonists. Psychopharmacology (Berl) 2007;193:159–170.
19 Provine RR: Yawning as a stereotyped action pattern and releasing stimulus. Ethology 1986;72:109–122.
20 Provine RR: Contagious yawning and infant imitation. B Psychonomic Soc 1989;27:125–126.
21 Rizzolatti G, et al: Resonance behaviors and mirror neurons. Arch Ital Biol 1999;137:85–100.
22 Ferrari W, Gessa GL, Vargiu L: Behavioral effects induced by intracisternally injected ACTH and MSH. Ann N Y Acad Sci 1963;104:330–345.
23 Serra G, et al: Hypophysectomy prevents ACTH-induced yawning and penile erection in rats. Pharmacol Biochem Behav 1987;26:277–279.
24 Gessa GL, et al: Stretching and yawning movements after intracerebral injection of ACTH. Rev Can Biol 1967;26:229–236.
25 Argiolas A, et al: ACTH- and alpha-MSH-induced grooming, stretching, yawning and penile erection in male rats: site of action in the brain and role of melanocortin receptors. Brain Res Bull 2000;51:425–431.
26 Argiolas A, et al: Paraventricular nucleus lesion prevents yawning and penile erection induced by apomorphine and oxytocin but not by ACTH in rats. Brain Res 1987;421:349–352.
27 Argiolas A, Melis MR, Gessa GL: Yawning and penile erection: central dopamine-oxytocin-adrenocorticotropin connection. Ann NY Acad Sci 1988; 525:330–337.
28 Argiolas A, et al: d(CH2)5Tyr(Me)-[Orn8]vasotocin, a potent oxytocin antagonist, antagonizes penile erection and yawning induced by oxytocin and apomorphine, but not by ACTH-(1–24). Eur J Pharmacol 1987;134:221–224.
29 Urba-Holmgren R, Gonzalez RM, Holmgren B: Is yawning a cholinergic response? Nature 1977;267: 261–262.
30 Kimura H, et al: Role of adrenergic neuronal activity in the yawning induced by tacrine and NIK-247 in rats. Pharmacol Biochem Behav 1992;43:985–991.
31 Ogura H, et al: Central and peripheral activity of cholinesterase inhibitors as revealed by yawning and fasciculation in rats. Eur J Pharmacol 2001;415: 157–164.
32 Zarrindast MR, Poursoltan M: Interactions of drugs acting on central dopamine receptors and cholinoceptors on yawning responses in the rat induced by apomorphine, bromocriptine or physostigmine. Br J Pharmacol 1989;96:843–848.
33 Ushijima I, et al: Modification of apomorphine-, physostigmine- and pilocarpine-induced yawning after long-term treatment with neuroleptic or cholinergic agents. Arch Int Pharmacodyn Ther 1984; 271:180–188.
34 Yamada K, Furukawa T: Direct evidence for involvement of dopaminergic inhibition and cholinergic activation in yawning. Psychopharmacology (Berl) 1980;67:39–43.
35 Fujikawa M, et al: The new muscarinic M_1-receptor agonist YM796 evokes yawning and increases oxytocin secretion from the posterior pituitary gland in rats. Pharmacol Biochem Behav 1996;55:55–60.
36 Fujikawa M, et al: Involvement of beta-adrenoceptors in regulation of the yawning induced by neuropeptides, oxytocin and alpha-melanocyte-stimulating hormone, in rats. Pharmacol Biochem Behav 1995; 50:339–343.

37 Gower AJ: Effects of acetylcholine agonists and antagonists on yawning and analgesia in the rat. Eur J Pharmacol 1987;139:79–89.
38 Wood PL, et al: Increase of hippocampal acetylcholine turnover rate and the stretching-yawning syndrome elicited by alpha-MSH and ACTH. Life Sci 1978;22:673–678.
39 Argiolas A, Melis MR, Gessa GL: Oxytocin: an extremely potent inducer of penile erection and yawning in male rats. Eur J Pharmacol 1986;130:265–272.
40 Collins GT, et al: Dopamine Agonist-Induced Yawning in Rats: A Dopamine D3 Receptor-Mediated Behavior. J Pharmacol Exp Ther 2005;314:310–319.
41 Melis MR, Stancampiano R, Argiolas A: Hippocampal oxytocin mediates apomorphine-induced penile erection and yawning. Pharmacol Biochem Behav 1992;42:61–66.
42 Melis MR, Argiolas A, Gessa GL: Oxytocin-induced penile erection and yawning: site of action in the brain. Brain Res 1986;398:259–265.
43 Melis MR, Argiolas A, Gessa GL: Evidence that apomorphine induces penile erection and yawning by releasing oxytocin in the central nervous system. Eur J Pharmacol 1989;164:565–570.
44 Melis MR, Stancampiano R, Argiolas A: Penile erection and yawning induced by paraventricular NMDA injection in male rats are mediated by oxytocin. Pharmacol Biochem Behav 1994;48:203–207.
45 Melis MR, et al: Effect of apomorphine on oxytocin concentrations in different brain areas and plasma of male rats. Eur J Pharmacol 1990;182:101–107.
46 Melis MR, Argiolas A: Role of central nitric oxide in the control of penile erection and yawning. Prog Neuropsychopharmacol Biol Psychiatry 1997;21:899–922.
47 Melis MR, Argiolas A: Nitric oxide donors induce penile erection and yawning when injected in the central nervous system of male rats. Eur J Pharmacol 1995;294:1–9.
48 Melis MR, et al: Nitroglycerin-induced penile erection and yawning in male rats: mechanism of action in the brain. Brain Res Bull 1995;36:527–531.
49 Melis MR, Argiolas A: Nitric oxide synthase inhibitors prevent apomorphine- and oxytocin-induced penile erection and yawning in male rats. Brain Res Bull 1993;32:71–74.
50 Melis MR, Stancampiano R, Argiolas A: Prevention by NG-nitro-L-arginine methyl ester of apomorphine- and oxytocin-induced penile erection and yawning: site of action in the brain. Pharmacol Biochem Behav 1994;48:799–804.
51 Melis MR, Argiolas A: Reduction of drug-induced yawning and penile erection and of noncontact erections in male rats by the activation of GABAA receptors in the paraventricular nucleus: involvement of nitric oxide. Eur J Neurosci 2002;15:852–860.
52 Melis MR, Succu S, Argiolas A: Dopamine agonists increase nitric oxide production in the paraventricular nucleus of the hypothalamus: correlation with penile erection and yawning. Eur J Neurosci 1996;8:2056–2063.
53 Melis MR, Stancampiano R, Argiolas A: Role of nitric oxide in penile erection and yawning induced by 5-HT1c receptor agonists in male rats. Naunyn Schmiedebergs Arch Pharmacol 1995;351:439–445.
54 Poggioli R, et al: Nitric oxide is involved in the ACTH-induced behavioral syndrome. Peptides 1995;16:1263–1268.
55 Mogilnicka E, Klimek V: Drugs affecting dopamine neurons and yawning behavior. Pharmacol Biochem Behav 1977;7:303–305.
56 Dubuc I, et al: Antagonism of the apomorphine-induced yawning by 'atypical' neuroleptics. Neuropharmacology 1982;21:1203–1206.
57 Holmgren B, Urba-Holmgren R: Interaction of cholinergic and dopaminergic influences on yawning behavior. Acta Neurobiol Exp (Wars) 1980;40:633–642.
58 Stahle L, Ungerstedt U: Assessment of dopamine autoreceptor agonist properties of apomorphine, (+)-3-PPP and (-)-3-PPP by recording of yawning behaviour in rats. Eur J Pharmacol 1984;98:307–310.
59 Dourish CT, Cooper SJ, Philips SR: Yawning elicited by systemic and intrastriatal injection of piribedil and apomorphine in the rat. Psychopharmacology (Berl) 1985;86:175–181.
60 Yamada K, et al: Involvement of septal and striatal dopamine D-2 receptors in yawning behavior in rats. Psychopharmacology (Berl) 1986;90:9–13.
61 Melis MR, Argiolas A, Gessa GL: Apomorphine-induced penile erection and yawning: site of action in brain. Brain Res 1987;415:98–104.
62 Urba-Holmgren R, Holmgren B, Anias J: Pre- and post-synaptic dopaminergic receptors involved in apomorphine-induced yawning. Acta Neurobiol Exp (Wars) 1982;42:115–125.
63 Yamada K, et al: Possible involvement of differing classes of dopamine D-2 receptors in yawning and stereotypy in rats. Psychopharmacology (Berl) 1990;100:141–144.
64 Stahle L: Do autoreceptors mediate dopamine agonist–induced yawning and suppression of exploration? A critical review. Psychopharmacology (Berl) 1992;106:1–13.

65 Stahle L, Ungerstedt U: Reduction of extracellular dopamine levels can be dissociated from suppression of exploratory behaviour in rats. Acta Physiol Scand 1987;130:533–534.

66 Stahle L, Ungerstedt U: Yawning and suppression of exploration in amphetamine-treated rats, incompatibility with the autoreceptor hypothesis. Psychopharmacology (Berl) 1989;97:553–560.

67 Stahle L, Ungerstedt U: Discrepancy in the time course of EMD 23448 induced yawning and reduction of extracellular dopamine. Psychopharmacology (Berl) 1989;97:275–276.

68 Stahle L, Ungerstedt U: Yawning and suppression of exploration induced by dopamine agonists: no relation to extracellular striatal levels of dopamine. Pharmacol Biochem Behav 1990;35:201–209.

69 Collins GT, et al: Proerectile effects of dopamine D2-like agonists are mediated by the D3 receptor in rats and mice. J Pharmacol Exp Ther 2009;329:210–217.

70 Baladi MG, Newman AH, France CP: Dopamine D3 receptors mediate the discriminative stimulus effects of quinpirole in free-feeding rats. J Pharmacol Exp Ther 2009.

71 Collins GT, et al: Food restriction alters pramipexole-induced yawning, hypothermia, and locomotor activity in rats: Evidence for sensitization of dopamine D2 receptor-mediated effects. J Pharmacol Exp Ther 2008.

72 Collins GT, Woods JH: Drug and Reinforcement History as Determinants of the Response-Maintaining Effects of Quinpirole in the Rat. J Pharmacol Exp Ther 2007;323:599–605.

73 Roeling TA, et al: Behavioural effects of NMDA injected into the hypothalamic paraventricular nucleus of the rat. Brain Res 1991;550:220–224.

74 Melis MR, Stancampiano R, Argiolas A: Effect of excitatory amino acid receptor antagonists on apomorphine-, oxytocin- and ACTH-induced penile erection and yawning in male rats. Eur J Pharmacol 1992;220:43–48.

75 Melis MR, Stancampiano R, Argiolas A: Nitric oxide synthase inhibitors prevent N-methyl-D-aspartic acid-induced penile erection and yawning in male rats. Neurosci Lett 1994;179:9–12.

76 Melis MR, et al: N-methyl-D-aspartic acid-induced penile erection and yawning: role of hypothalamic paraventricular nitric oxide. Eur J Pharmacol 1997; 328:115–123.

77 Urba-Holmgren R, et al: Serotonergic modulation of yawning. Pharmacol Biochem Behav 1979;11:371–372.

78 Berendsen HH, Jenck F, Broekkamp CL: Involvement of 5-HT1C-receptors in drug-induced penile erections in rats. Psychopharmacology (Berl) 1990;101: 57–61.

79 Stancampiano R, Melis MR, Argiolas A: Penile erection and yawning induced by 5-HT1C receptor agonists in male rats: relationship with dopaminergic and oxytocinergic transmission. Eur J Pharmacol 1994;261:149–155.

80 Protais P, et al: Post-synaptic 5-HT1A receptor involvement in yawning and penile erections induced by apomorphine, physostigmine and mCPP in rats. Psychopharmacology (Berl) 1995;120: 376–383.

81 Matsumoto S, et al: Potentiation by serotonergic inhibition of yawning induced by dopamine receptor agonists in rats. Pharmacol Biochem Behav 1989;32:815–818.

82 Okuyama S, et al: Relation between yawning behavior and central serotonergic neuronal system in rats. Naunyn Schmiedebergs Arch Pharmacol 1987;335: 667–672.

83 Simon P, et al: 5-HT1A receptor agonists prevent in rats the yawning and penile erections induced by direct dopamine agonists. Psychopharmacology (Berl) 1992;108:47–50.

84 Fratta W, et al: Reciprocal antagonism between ACTH1–24 and beta-endorphin in rats. Neurosci Lett 1981;24:71–74.

85 Vergoni AV, et al: Tolerance develops to the behavioural effects of ACTH-(1–24) during continuous i.c.v. infusion in rats, and is associated with increased hypothalamic levels of beta-endorphin. Neuropeptides 1989;14:93–98.

86 Melis MR, et al: Prevention by morphine of apomorphine- and oxytocin-induced penile erection and yawning: site of action in the brain. Neuropsychopharmacology 1992;6:17–21.

87 Melis MR, Succu S, Argiolas A: Prevention by morphine of N-methyl-D-aspartic acid-induced penile erection and yawning: involvement of nitric oxide. Brain Res Bull 1997;44:689–694.

88 Melis MR, et al: Prevention by morphine of apomorphine- and oxytocin-induced penile erection and yawning: involvement of nitric oxide. Naunyn Schmiedebergs Arch Pharmacol 1997;355:595–600.

89 Zarrindast MR, Jamshidzadeh A: Inhibitory effect of morphine on yawning induced by cholinoceptor and dopamine D2 receptor activation in rats. Br J Pharmacol 1992;105:675–678.

90 Zharkovsky A, et al: Role of dopamine receptors in the dual effect of naloxone on quinpirole-induced yawning in morphine pretreated rats. Naunyn Schmiedebergs Arch Pharmacol 1993;347:478–482.

91 Himmelsbach CK: Studies of certain addiction characteristics of (a) dihydromorphine ('paramorphan'), (b) dihydrodesoxymorphine-D ('desomorphine'), (c) dihydrodesoxycodeine-D ('desocodeine'), and (d) methyldihydromorphinone ('metopon'). J Pharmacol Exp Ther 1939;67:239–249.
92 Seevers MH: Opiate addiction in the monkey I. Methods of study. J Pharmacol Exp Ther 1936;56: 147–156.
93 Zharkovsky A, et al: Concurrent nimodipine attenuates the withdrawal signs and the increase of cerebral dihydropyridine binding after chronic morphine treatment in rats. Naunyn Schmiedebergs Arch Pharmacol 1993;347:483–486.
94 Doger E, et al: GABAergic modulation of yawning behavior. Pharmacol Biochem Behav 1989;34:237–240.
95 Zarrindast MR, Toloui V, Hashemi B: Effects of GABAergic drugs on physostigmine-induced yawning in rats. Psychopharmacology (Berl) 1995;122: 297–300.
96 Melis MR, et al: Activation of gamma-aminobutyric acid(A) receptors in the paraventricular nucleus of the hypothalamus reduces apomorphine-, N-methyl-D-aspartic acid- and oxytocin-induced penile erection and yawning in male rats. Neurosci Lett 2000; 281:127–130.
97 Nava F, et al: gamma-Hydroxybutyric acid and baclofen decrease extracellular acetylcholine levels in the hippocampus via GABA(B) receptors. Eur J Pharmacol 2001;430:261–263.
98 Ferrari F, Giuliani D: Influence of idazoxan on the dopamine D2 receptor agonist-induced behavioural effects in rats. Eur J Pharmacol 1993;250:51–57.
99 Mogilnicka E, Boissard CG, Delini-Stula A: Effects of apomorphine, TL-99 and 3-PPP on yawning in rats. Neuropharmacology 1984;23:19–22.
100 Gower AJ, Berendsen HH, Broekkamp CL: Antagonism of drug-induced yawning and penile erections in rats. Eur J Pharmacol 1986;122:239–244.
101 Zarrindast MR, et al: Influence of different adrenoceptor agonists and antagonists on physostigmine-induced yawning in rats. Pharmacol Biochem Behav 1999;62:1–5.
102 Baladi MG, France CP: High fat diet and food restriction differentially modify the behavioral effects of quinpirole and raclopride in rats. Eur J Pharmacol 2009;610:55–60.
103 Chen J, et al: Design, synthesis, and evaluation of potent and selective ligands for the dopamine 3 (D3) receptor with a novel in vivo behavioral profile. J Med Chem 2008;51:5905–5908.
104 Sevak RJ, et al: Insulin replacement restores the behavioral effects of quinpirole and raclopride in streptozotocin-treated rats. J Pharmacol Exp Ther 2007;320:1216–1223.

Gregory T. Collins
Department of Pharmacology, University of Michigan
1301 MSRB III, 1150 W. Medical Center Dr.
Ann Arbor, MI 48109 (USA)
Tel. +1 734 764 2307, Fax +1 734 764 7118, E-Mail collinsg@umich.edu

Walusinski O (ed): The Mystery of Yawning in Physiology and Disease.
Front Neurol Neurosci. Basel, Karger, 2010, vol 28, pp 107–112

Yawn, Yawn, Yawn, Yawn; Yawn, Yawn, Yawn! The Social, Evolutionary and Neuroscientific Facets of Contagious Yawning

Steven M. Platek

Georgia Gwinnett College, Lawrenceville, Ga., USA

Abstract

Contagious yawning is a common phenomenon affecting upwards of 60% of healthy humans. It has also been observed, at a lesser rate, in great apes and other primates. Here I summarize the suggestion that contagious yawning is a primitive expression of social cognition, namely empathy. Susceptibility to contagious yawning is correlated with the speed in recognizing one's own face, theory of mind processing, and is also associated with activation in regions of the brain that have been associated with social cognitive processes. This suggests that contagious yawning may be an evolutionarily old process that begot a higher level of social cognition in certain species.

Did you just yawn? The title of this chapter was designed in such a way as to evoke a common human behavioral response, i.e. to yawn contagiously. If you did yawn, you are among 60% of other humans that also respond contagiously to hearing, seeing, observing and even reading about yawning [1–3].

While contagious yawning is a common experience among people, yawning actually remains one of the great understudied phenomena of science. You might mistakenly believe that we yawn to reset the balance of blood oxygenation; however, this is not actually the case. It turns out that yawning may serve a more adaptive function: cooling the brain [4–6]. The function of yawning is not, however, the focus of this chapter. Here I will discuss the current evidence that contagious yawning is a byproduct of evolutionarily designed programs related to empathy, social cognition and/or self-awareness.

Relationship between Self-Awareness and Other Awareness

In 1970, Gallup [7] discovered that chimpanzees possess the ability to recognize themselves in a mirror [see also: 8–15]. He suggested that the now infamous mirror test was a marker for the presence of a sense of self-awareness. Furthermore, combining his findings with evidence that was emerging from cognitive primatology, he hypothesized that the ability to generalize about mental states – mental state attribution – presupposed a sense of self-awareness. He theorized that the presence of self-awareness paved the way for a cognitive substrate for mental state attribution, or theory of mind. The possession of a theory of mind lends to it the ability to empathize, sympathize, relate emotionally to another individual, anthropomorphize, and generally experience the world through another person's perspective. Interestingly, many of us do not have to 'think' about theory of mind, i.e. for most healthy humans the ability to think about another person's mental state is automatic.

In this respect, when we observe another person experiencing something, we have an inherent experience that is similar to that person. However, in most cases we do not automatically emulate that person's experience. Let me provide an example. If I were to walk across the stage in the front of one of my classrooms and trip over an electric wire that was laying in my way. The audience would be in a position to empathize with my position and experience. They might, admittedly, find humor in my ostensibly embarrassing behavior. And that would be an appropriate mental state attribution. They would be utilizing their experience with non-fatal falls which is highly correlated with a feeling or cognitive experience of embarrassment. However, if after a few seconds of laughing they discovered that upon tripping over the cable I had landed face down on the stage and there was a pool of red liquid forming quickly around my head, (I hope) their chuckles would turn to worry. They would be able to see that my fall was much more serious than they had originally conceptualized. They would not have to 'think' actively about this change in cognition, rather because our brains are hard-wired for sociality there is little actual thinking necessary for this process to take place. In the previous example, onlookers would have to be able to rapidly change inference about my mental state to make an adaptive response (albeit in my favor) to call for emergency help. They would not need to cognate about the decision: 'He seems to have tripped. That was funny in my past, and so it must be funny now. Oh wait, he's fallen on his face and is bleeding. I need a new cognition for that …' If our empathic understanding of others' mental states were to flow in this fashion, we would all be pretty socially awkward!

All that being said, in neither of these cases would the audience's empathic mental state attribution result in an actual replication of my experience in an observer. The audience would not spontaneously feel embarrassed and then upon falling on my face get sudden feeling of panic and pain and fear! Their feelings are attributions, good guesses, hypotheses about how I might be feeling or what my experience is like. In certain cases, the attribution produces a contagion. This typically occurs in the context of a personal emotional experience such as someone crying. If your sister, mother, child or even close friend came to your house and started to cry and express extreme sadness you might be compelled, somewhat uncontrollably, to begin crying yourself. Your empathic understanding of her mental state has manifested itself in your own outward expression. Similar examples exist in the realm of happiness; in fact, laughter is quite contagious. Coughing may also be contagious. Even these attributions turned experiences are somewhat controllable. When you child comes running into your arms crying one can, if they try hard enough, usually quell the crying response. In the case of contagious yawning, however, once the onset of a yawn begins it is virtually impossible to quell the execution of the yawn.

The evidence for the relationship between self-processing and mental state attribution comes from comparative primatology, developmental psychology, cognitive psychology and cognitive neuroscience. I have briefly summarized the major findings here. First, since the discovery that chimpanzees could recognize themselves in a mirror, there have been numerous studies aimed at testing whether chimpanzees (and other great apes) have the capacity for a theory of mind [8, 14, 16]. Similarly, correlate tasks have been made on other species including but not limited to corvids, elephants, cetaceans, and lesser primates. In fact, it seems like only those species that reliably demonstrate a sense of self-awareness also show a corresponding capacity for other-awareness.

Developmental psychology represents another example of this. Children tend to develop a sense of self at about 15 months of age [8]. During this time, they begin to use personal pronouns and referential pointing. It is also during this time that children show the ability to recognize themselves in a mirror. Amsterdam [17] first tested this by converting the mark test, used in non-human primates, into the rouge test. It is important to note that shortly after the emergence of self-awareness, or more specifically mirror self-recognition, children begin to develop theory of mind. That is, shortly after 15–24 months of age – when children show mirror self-recognition – they begin to develop a set of cognitions based on desire, belief and social relationships.

When it comes to adult cognition, a similar relationship exists. Keenan et al. [18–23] were the first to test for reaction time differences in self-face recognition. He and his team showed that people were significantly faster at differentiating self-faces from other faces when using their left-hand. This he interpreted as an indication for a right hemisphere bias for self-processing. As a follow-up to Keenan's studies, Platek et al. [24, 25] replicated the left-hand/right hemisphere bias for self-processing and also showed that reaction times to self-face correlated with performance on higher level theory of mind tasks. In an fMRI study, Platek et al. [26] showed that the same regions of the right frontal lobe were recruited when participants were asked to recognize their own face and when they were asked to solve a theory of mind task. Several other studies have now also supported the link between self-processing and theory of mind by using a plethora of methodological techniques, including reaction times and functional neuroimaging.

Contagious Yawning in the Self-Other Relationship

Because contagious yawning produces an unconsciously controlled automatic release of a contagious yawn in an observer – several researchers, e.g. Platek et al. [2, 3] have hypothesized that contagious yawning might be an evolutionary predecessor to a more sophisticated sense of empathy/mental state attribution. In order to test this, Platek et al. [2] investigated whether there was a relationship between speed in identifying one's own face, performance on a set of theory of mind stories, and susceptibility to contagious yawning. They showed that people who were better at solving higher order theory of mind (faux pas) tasks were more susceptible to contagious yawning. They interpreted these findings as showing a link between the automatic empathic processing associated with contagious yawning and other theory of mind processes. Taken together with the finding that theory of mind and self-processing share neural architecture, this indicates that self-processing, theory of mind and contagious yawning might share similar substrates as well as similar processing.

Evidence from Neuroimaging

There are now a handful of studies incorporating functional neuroimaging to investigate the neural substrates associated with contagious yawning. The first of these was by Platek et al. [3]. They showed activation in posterior midline substrates – the precuneus and posterior cingulate. Schurmann et al. [27] conducted a similar study and demonstrated activation in the superior temporal sulcus and more general activation across a mirror neuron system. Two studies [28, 29] found activation in frontal lobe circuitry. While Platek et al. [3] argued that activation of the posterior cingulate/precuneous was associated with autobiographical memories and self-processing, this finding might appear to be difficult to rectify in the presence of such disparate findings from other laboratories. However, if we inspect each of the findings from the various fMRI studies of contagious yawning, a commonality exists: each study shows activation in cortical association areas that have been indirectly linked to theory of mind and/or self-processing. Thus, if one takes these early and inconclusive findings from functional neuroimaging in conjunction with the cognitive and behavioral expressions of contagious yawning within and between species, the argument for contagious yawning being a product of primitive/vestigial empathic drives stands firm.

Conclusions

The expression of contagious yawing appears to be relatively robust in man and partially present in lesser primates. Contagious yawning appears to exist in species that also show a capacity for self-processing and theory of mind, albeit rudimentary in some cases. Recent neuroimaging evidence suggests that there could be multiple brain loci involved in the contagious yawning response; however, it's important to note that each fMRI study has identified activation in brain substrates that have been implicated in social cognition, self-processing and/or theory of mind in other studies. Thus, it is our contention that contagious yawning is a vestigial fixed action pattern that may be a glimpse into the neurobiological substrates that gave rise to more sophisticated social cognitive processes such as theory of mind.

References

1 Lehman HE: Yawning: a homeostatic reflex and its psychological significance. Bull Meninger Clin 1979;43:123–136.

2 Platek SM, Critton SR, Myers TE, Gallup GG: Contagious yawning: the role of self-awareness and mental state attribution. Brain Res Cogn Brain Res 2003;17:223–227.

3 Platek SM, Mohamed FB, Gallup GG Jr: Contagious yawning and the brain. Brain Res Cogn Brain Res 2005;23:448–452.

4 Gallup AC, Gallup GG Jr: Yawning and thermoregulation. Physiol Behav 2008;95:10–16.

5 Gallup AC, Gallup GG Jr: Medical implications of excessive yawning in relation to thermoregulatory dysfunction. Eur J Neurol 2009;16:e120.

6 Gallup AC, Gallup GG Jr: Venlafaxine-induced excessive yawning: a thermoregulatory connection. Prog Neuropsychopharmacol Biol Psychiatry 2009; 33:747.

7 Gallup GG Jr: Chimpanzees: self-recognition. Science 1970;167:86–87.

8 Anderson JR: The development of self-recognition: a review. Dev Psychobiol 1984;17:35–49.

9 Anderson JR: Self-recognition in dolphins: credible cetaceans; compromised criteria, controls, and conclusions. Conscious Cogn 1995;4:239–243.

10 Anderson JR, Gallup GG Jr: Self-recognition in Saguinus? A critical essay. Anim Behav 1997;54: 1563–1567.

11 Gallup GG Jr: Absence of self-recognition in a monkey (Macaca fascicularis) following prolonged exposure to a mirror. Dev Psychobiol 1977;10:281–284.

12 Gallup GG Jr: Do minds exist in species other than our own? Neurosci Biobehav Rev 1985;9:631–641.

13 Gallup GG Jr: Mirrors, minds, and cetaceans. Conscious Cogn 1995;4:226–228.

14 Gallup GG Jr: On the rise and fall of self-conception in primates. Ann N Y Acad Sci 1997;818:72–82.

15 Gallup GG Jr, Wallnau LB, Suarez SD: Failure to find self-recognition in mother-infant and infant-infant rhesus monkey pairs. Folia Primatol (Basel) 1980;33:210–219.

16 de Veer MW, Gallup GG Jr, Theall LA, van den Bos R, Povinelli DJ: An 8-year longitudinal study of mirror self-recognition in chimpanzees (Pan troglodytes). Neuropsychologia 2003;41:229–234.

17 Amsterdam B: Mirror self-image reactions before the age of two. Dev Psychobiol 1972;5:297–305.

18 Keenan JP, McCutcheon B, Freund S, Gallup GG Jr, Sanders G, Pascual-Leone A: Left hand advantage in a self-face recognition task. Neuropsychologia 1999;37:1421–1425.

19 Keenan JP, Ganis G, Freund S, Pascual-Leone A: Self-face identification is increased with left hand responses. Laterality 2000;5:259–268.

20 Keenan JP, Wheeler M, Platek SM, Lardi G, Lassonde M: Self-face processing in a callosotomy patient. Eur J Neurosci 2003;18:2391–2395.

21 Keenan JP, Rubio J, Racioppi C, Johnson A, Barnacz A: The right hemisphere and the dark side of consciousness. Cortex 2005;41:695–704, discussion 731–734.

22 Keenan JP, Nelson AM, Pascual-Leone A: Self-recognition and the right hemisphere. Nature 2001; 409:305.

23 Keenan JP, Wheeler M, Gallup GG Jr, Pascual-Leone A: Self-awareness and the right prefrontal cortex. Trends Cogn Sci 2000;4:338–344.

24 Platek SM, Myers TE, Critton SR, Gallup GG Jr: A left-hand advantage for self-description: the impact of schizotypal personality traits. Schizophr Res 2003;65:147–151.

25 Platek SM, Thomson JW, Gallup GG Jr: Cross-modal self-recognition: the role of visual, auditory, and olfactory primes. Conscious Cogn 2004;13:197–210.

26 Platek SM, Keenan JP, Gallup GG Jr, Mohamed FB: Where am I? The neurological correlates of self and other. Brain Res Cogn Brain Res 2004;19:114–122.
27 Schurmann M, Hesse MD, Stephan KE, Saarela M, Zilles K, Hari R, Fink GR: Yearning to yawn: the neural basis of contagious yawning. Neuroimage 2005;24:1260–1264.
28 Arnott SR, Singhal A, Goodale MA: An investigation of auditory contagious yawning. Cogn Affect Behav Neurosci 2009;9:335–342.
29 Nahab FB, Hattori N, Saad ZS, Hallett M: Contagious yawning and the frontal lobe: an fMRI study. Hum Brain Mapp 2009;30:1744–1751.

Steven M. Platek
Associate Professor of Psychology, Georgia Gwinnett College
Lawrenceville, GA 30043 (USA)
Tel. +1 404 734 1023, E-Mail splatek@gmail.com

Walusinski O (ed): The Mystery of Yawning in Physiology and Disease.
Front Neurol Neurosci. Basel, Karger, 2010, vol 28, pp 113–119

Developmental and Comparative Perspectives of Contagious Yawning

Atsushi Senju

Birkbeck College, University of London, London, UK

Abstract

Contagious yawning (i.e. yawning triggered by perceiving others' yawning) is a well-documented phenomenon, but the mechanism underlying it is still unclear. In this chapter, I review the current evidence about: (1) developmental studies with typically and atypically developing populations, and (2) comparative studies in non-human animals. Developmental studies have revealed that contagious yawning is disturbed in individuals with autism spectrum disorders, suggesting that contagious yawning may share a developmental basis with the capacity for theory of mind. Comparative studies have suggested that contagious yawning can be observed in non-primate species, such as domestic dogs. As dogs are known to have exceptional skills in communicating with humans, it has also been suggested that contagious yawning may be related to the capacity for social communication. These results from developmental and comparative studies are consistent with the claim that the mechanism underlying contagious yawning relates to the capacity for empathy.

Contagious yawning (i.e. yawning triggered by perceiving others' yawning) is a well-documented phenomenon. Previous studies have consistently reported that, in a naturalistic or controlled experimental context, 45–60% of human adults yawn when they observe, hear or imagine others' yawning [1]. This is not due to common environmental factors between two yawners, such as temperature, lighting or the lack of oxygen, because pre-recorded yawning video clips and sounds can also induce contagious yawning [2–4]. Recently, this phenomenon has attracted a great deal of attention in the fields of developmental and comparative cognitive sciences. Apart from the intrinsic interest in this well-known but puzzling phenomenon, its attraction has been due to the fact that it is apparently empathetic: the observation of the emotional or physiological status of other individuals affects the emotional or physiological status of observer in a corresponding manner. Some researchers claim that the presence of contagious yawning in non-human animals is an index for their capacity for empathy [5, 6] and absence of contagious yawning in a developmental disorder or a psychiatric condition suggests a disturbance in their capacity for empathy [7, 8].

In this chapter, I review the current evidence from: (1) developmental studies with typically and atypically developing populations, and (2) comparative studies in non-human animals, discuss implications for the mechanism underlying contagious yawning, and raise several issues for future studies.

Typical and Atypical Development of Contagious Yawning

Apart from the initial case study by Piaget [9] – who, from observing his own daughter, reported that yawning in response to seeing a yawn started in the second year of life – Anderson and Meno [2] are the first and the only researchers to report a developmental trajectory of contagious yawning from an elaborate cross-sectional study. In their study, typically developing children aged 2–11 years old were exposed to a video presentation of yawning adults and a story including a yawning protagonist. The results revealed that some of the children aged 5 years or older showed contagious yawning in response to the video stimuli, and some of the children aged 6 years or older showed yawning in response to the yawning story. These results failed to replicate this early observation by Piaget [9], but the negative results reported for preschoolers should be treated with caution. For example, Anderson and Meno [2] discussed the possibility that familiarity with yawning adults may be relevant to the differences between these two studies.

In addition to the investigation of typical development, other scientists, including our group, have investigated the development of contagious yawning in children with autism spectrum disorders (ASD), who show atypical development in social interaction and communication [10]. Firstly, our research group has presented videotaped yawning as well as control mouth-opening actions to children with ASD as well as typically developing children between the ages of 7 and 15 years old [8]. Typically developing children showed more yawning in response to yawning movies than to control movies. By contrast, children with ASD showed equally frequent yawning in response to both yawning and control movies (fig. 1). These results replicated those of Anderson and Meno [2] in that typically developing children at the age of 7 years or older show contagious yawning. More importantly, this was the first study to demonstrate the absence of contagious yawning in children with ASD. Secondly, Giganti and Esposito Ziello [11] further explored the impact of the level of intellectual development upon the tendency to yawn contagion in children with ASD, by comparing children with ASD with higher and lower intellectual ability between the ages of 11 and 15 years old. They also used the auditory stimuli of yawning sounds, in addition to the visual stimuli of a yawning face, and also had the frequency of spontaneous yawning recorded by the parents. The results replicated the finding that both visual

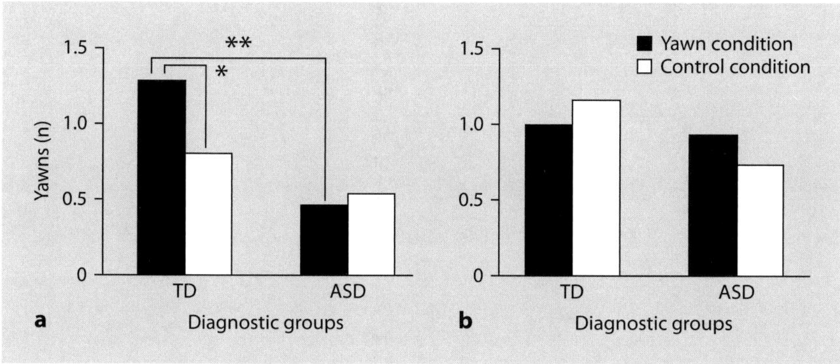

Fig. 1. Average frequency of yawns in participants during or after yawn and control conditions in Senju et al. [8] (**a**) and in Senju et al. [12] (**b**). TD = Typically developing children. ** $p < 0.01$; * $p < 0.05$. Reproduced with permission.

and auditory yawning stimuli elicited more yawning in typically developing children than in children with ASD. They did not find any effect of intellectual ability or group differences in the frequency of spontaneous yawning. These two studies suggest that children with ASD have an impairment in the mechanism relevant to the capacity for contagious yawning.

Thirdly, a recent study by the author's group [12] used a similar task used in Senju et al. [8] with an additional instruction to fixate on the eyes of the yawning face. The aim of this study was to test the hypothesis that an absence of contagious yawning in ASD is related to atypical social orienting, particularly the reduced spontaneous fixation on the eyes [13], because it has been reported that yawning eyes are as potent stimuli in eliciting yawning as the whole face, but a yawning mouth alone is not [14]. The results revealed that children with ASD yawned equally frequently in response to yawning stimuli as typically developing children once the additional instruction to fixate on the eyes was added. This is consistent with the hypothesis that reduced spontaneous fixations on the eyes may contribute to the absence of contagious yawning in ASD.

This research is consistent with the claim that the mechanism underlying contagious yawning relates to the capacity for theory of mind [4], the impairment of which is widely and consistently reported in individuals with ASD [15, 16]. However, the preliminary results of Senju et al. [12] may suggest that the absence of contagious yawning in ASD is mediated by the atypical pattern of spontaneous orienting to the eyes [13], not by the impairment in theory of mind per se. It is also possible that atypical social orienting is the common developmental basis of both atypical contagious yawning and the difficulty in theory of mind [17]. Further studies will be required to test the early development of contagious yawning in ASD, and its relation to the development of the social brain network.

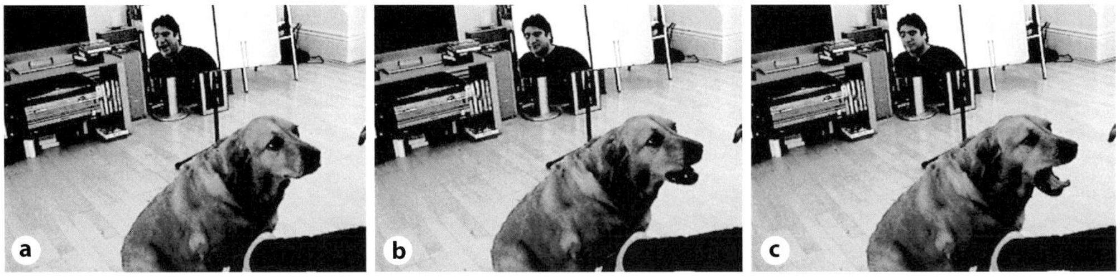

Fig. 2. A yawn response during the presentation of a human yawn. The experimenter's face can be seen at the top of each image, which was recorded in the mirror placed behind the dog. The dog observed the experimenter yawning (**a**), started yawning as the experimenter finished yawning (**b**) and then completed yawning (**c**). Reproduced with permission from Joly-Mascheroni et al. [6].

Contagious Yawning in Non-Human Animals

To the best of my knowledge, Anderson et al. [5] were the first to report quantitative data on contagious yawning in non-human animals. They presented yawning and control movies to 3 adult and 3 young chimpanzees *(Pan troglodytes)*, and found a significant increase in the frequency of yawning in response to yawning movies in 2 adult chimpanzees. This result was replicated by a larger follow-up study [18]. In addition, Paukner and Anderson [19] reported that yawning movies elicit more yawning than control movies in stumptail macaques *(Macaca arctoides)*. These studies suggest that the susceptibility to contagious yawning is not specific to humans, but could be shared with other non-human primate species.

A further question arises as to whether contagious yawning emerged during primate evolution, or is shared with an even wider range of animal species. To tackle this question, our research group conducted an experimental study to test whether domestic dogs *(Canis familiaris)* also show contagious yawning [6]. This study was motivated by several anecdotes from colleagues and other dog owners indicating their yawns elicit yawns from their dogs. Similar anecdotes can also be found in literature [20, 21]. In our study, 29 dogs observed a live presentation of acted yawns by an experimenter, as well as the same human experimenter's non-yawning mouth movement. The experimenter called the dogs and/or presented a small piece of bait in front of the experimenter's face to make sure that the dogs made clear eye contact with the experimenter just before the experimenter presented a yawning or control mouth movement. Testing was conducted in places familiar to each dog, between 11 am and 4 pm and after they had finished walking and had 1 of their 2 daily meals, to make sure that dogs attended the experiments in the least stressful way. In total, 21 out of 29 dogs yawned in response to the experimenter's yawns (fig. 2), but no dogs yawned in response to the control mouth movement produced by the same experimenter. These results clearly suggest that human yawns elicit a yawning response in dogs. Following our study, Harr et al. [22] presented video clips of humans and dogs yawning, as well as non-yawning mouth opening actions, to 15 dogs. Only 1 dog exhibited significantly more yawns in response to yawning video clips than to control video clips. It is not clear why Harr et al. [22] failed to replicate Joly-Mascheroni et al. [6], but it is likely that the way stimuli were presented contributed to the apparent discrepancy: it is possible that either the live presentation of stimuli, the social interaction between the yawning person and the dog, and/or establishment of eye contact before stimulus presentation is important for eliciting contagious yawning in dogs.

These results clearly demonstrated that human yawns elicit yawning in dogs, supporting the claim that the capacity for contagious yawning can be shared beyond the primate species. However, it is not necessarily warranted that the mechanism underlying contagious yawning is also shared among these species. For example, Paukner and Anderson [19] raised the possibility that apparently contagious yawning in stumptail macaques may be based on the heightened tension or stress induced by the observation of yawning, as yawning is a threatening signal in this species. Similarly, one could claim that part of the yawns observed in Joly-Mascheroni et al. [6] was a stress-related response induced by the yawning of a stranger, as some have argued that yawning in dogs is a response to acute stress [23]. However, more recent empirical studies [24, 25] have failed to confirm the relationship between stress and yawning, making this claim less convincing. Moreover, the presence of contagious yawning even when the potential 'tension yawns' were excluded from analyses [22] do not support this claim.

The current findings do not strictly support the relationship between theory of mind and contagious yawning, because there is no clear evidence supporting the presence of fully functional theory of mind in non-human animals, even in chimpanzees [26, 27]. However, this does not deny the possibility that a precursor of theory of mind may relate to the capacity for contagious yawning in these species. For example, dogs are sensitive to human attention and communication cues [28, 29], and may even infer the knowledge status of humans [30].

Conclusions and Future Directions

In this chapter, I have reviewed developmental and comparative studies of contagious yawning. Even though the scarcity of existing studies prevents us from drawing any firm conclusions, the current findings tend to suggest that contagious yawning shares its mechanism with the capacity for theory of mind. In particular, a series of studies on children with autism highlighted that spontaneous orientation to socially relevant stimuli such as eyes may mediate contagious yawning in humans and possibly in non-human animals. These suggestions from preliminary findings merit further investigation of the relationship between the development of social cognition and contagious yawning. In this final section, I will summarize some possible directions for future research.

Firstly, more studies are required to fully describe the developmental pathway of contagious yawning, as well as to assess the reasons behind the apparent contradiction between two of the existing developmental studies [2, 9] about the presence or absence of contagious yawning in children younger than 7 years. In addition, further studies are needed to test whether the absence of spontaneous contagious yawning is limited to children with autism, or can be observed in other developmental disorders that may or may not manifest impairments in social cognition.

Secondly, it is critical to test the prevalence of contagious yawning in non-human animals. As our recent study demonstrated the presence of contagious yawning in domestic dogs, it is possible that other non-primate species could also have the capacity for contagious yawning. Since our dog paper [6] was featured in the media, I have received numbers of anecdotes of yawn contagion from enthusiastic amateur naturalists and pet owners, including 4 independent reports about cats *(Felis catus)*, a report about horses *(Equus ferus caballus)*, an African grey parrot *(Psittacus erithacus)* and blackbirds *(Turdus merula)*, as well as a report about a failed attempt with foxes (exact species not known). Of course it is likely that these anecdotes are based on the over-interpretation of incidental episodes, but I still think it is worth investigating. At the same time, it is also important to study to what extent contagious yawning in non-human animals shares the mechanism with human yawn contagion.

Growing number of new reports have begun to shed light on the mechanism underlying contagious yawning and its relations to other cognitive mechanisms. Further studies in the neural, developmental and evolutionary origin of contagious yawning will help us to better understand the mechanism underlying yawning, as well as the mechanism underlying social interaction and communication.

Acknowledgments

The author was supported by a research fellowship (RES-063–27–0207) from the UK Economic and Social Research Council.

References

1 Provine RR: Yawning as a stereotyped action pattern and releasing stimulus. Ethology 1986;72:448–455.
2 Anderson JR, Meno P: Psychological influences on yawning in children. Curr Psychol Lett 2003;11. http://cpl.revues.org/index390.html.
3 Arnott SR, Singhal A, Goodale MA: An investigation of auditory contagious yawning. Cogn Affect Behav Neurosci 2009;9:335–342.
4 Platek SM, Critton SR, Myers TE, Gallup GG: Contagious yawning: the role of self-awareness and mental state attribution. Cogn Brain Res 2003;17:223–227.
5 Anderson JR, Myowa-Yamakoshi M, Matsuzawa T: Contagious yawning in chimpanzees. Proc R Soc B Biol Sci 2004;271:S468–S470.
6 Joly-Mascheroni RM, Senju A, Shepherd AJ: Dogs catch human yawns. Biol Lett 2008;4:446–448.

7 Haker H, Rössler W: Empathy in schizophrenia: impaired resonance. Eur Arch Psychiatry Clin Neurosci 2009;259:352–361.
8 Senju A, Maeda M, Kikuchi Y, Hasegawa T, Tojo Y, Osanai H: Absence of contagious yawning in children with autism spectrum disorder. Biol Lett 2007; 3:706–708.
9 Piaget J: Play, Dreams and Imitation in Childhood. London, Routledge & Kegan, 1951.
10 American Psychiatric Association: Diagnostic and Statistical Manual of Mental Disorders, ed 4 (text revision). Washington, APA, 2000.
11 Giganti F, Esposito Ziello M: Contagious and spontaneous yawning in autistic and typically developing children. Curr Psychol Lett 2009;25.
12 Senju A, Kikuchi Y, Akechi H, Hasegawa T, Tojo Y, Osanai H: Brief report: does eye contact induce contagious yawning in children with autism spectrum disorder? J Autism Dev Dis 2009;39:1598–1602.
13 Senju A, Johnson MH: Atypical eye contact in autism: models, mechanisms and development. Neurosci Biobehav Rev 2009;33:1204–1214.
14 Provine RR: Yawning and simulation science. Simulation 1989;53:193–194.
15 Baron-Cohen S, Leslie AM, Frith U: Does the autistic child have a 'theory of mind'? Cognition 1985;21:37–46.
16 Senju A, Southgate V, White S, Frith U: Mindblind eyes: an absence of spontaneous theory of mind in Asperger syndrome. Science 2009;325:883–885.
17 Senju A, Johnson MH: The eye contact effect: mechanisms and development. Trends Cogn Sci 2009;13: 127–134.
18 Campbell MW, Carter JD, Proctor D, Eisenberg ML, de Waal FBM: Computer animations stimulate contagious yawning in chimpanzees. Proc Biol Sci 2009; 276:4255–4259.
19 Paukner A, Anderson JR: Video-induced yawning in stumptail macaques (*Macaca arctoides*). Biol Lett 2006;2:36–38.
20 Dureau de la Malle A: Mémoire sur le développement des facultés intellectuelles des animaux sauvages et domestiqués. Ann Sci Nat 1831;21: 388–419.
21 Rugaas T: On Talking Terms with Dogs: Calming Signals. Wenatchee, Dogwise, 1997.
22 Harr A, Gilbert V, Phillips K: Do dogs (*Canis familiaris*) show contagious yawning? Anim Cogn 2009; 12:833–837.
23 Beerda B, Schilder MBH, van Hooff JARAM, de Vries HW, Mol JA: Behavioural, saliva cortisol and heart rate responses to different types of stimuli in dogs. Appl Anim Behav Sci 1998;58:365–381.
24 Hennessy MB, Morris A, Linden F: Evaluation of the effects of a socialization program in a prison on behavior and pituitary-adrenal hormone levels of shelter dogs. Appl Anim Behav Sci 2006;99:157–171.
25 Rooney NJ, Gaines SA, Bradshaw JWS: Behavioural and glucocorticoid responses of dogs (*Canis familiaris*) to kennelling: investigating mitigation of stress by prior habituation. Physiol Behav 2007;92: 847–854.
26 Call J, Tomasello M: Does the chimpanzee have a theory of mind? 30 years later. Trends Cogn Sci 2008;12:187–192.
27 Penn DC, Povinelli DJ: On the lack of evidence that non-human animals possess anything remotely resembling a 'theory of mind'. Philos Trans R Soc B Biol Sci 2007;362:731–744.
28 Hare B, Brown M, Williamson C, Tomasello M: The domestication of social cognition in dogs. Science 2002;298:1634–1636.
29 Topal J, Gergely G, Erdohegyi A, Csibra G, Miklosi A: Differential sensitivity to human communication in dogs, wolves, and human infants. Science 2009; 325:1269–1272.
30 Virányi Z, Topál J, Miklósi Á, Csányi V: A nonverbal test of knowledge attribution: a comparative study on dogs and children. Anim Cogn 2006;9:13–26.

Atsushi Senju
Centre for Brain and Cognitive Development, Birkbeck
University of London, Malet Street
London WC1E 7HX (UK)
Tel. +44 207 631 6895, Fax +44 207 631 6587, E-Mail a.senju@bbk.ac.uk

Walusinski O (ed): The Mystery of Yawning in Physiology and Disease.
Front Neurol Neurosci. Basel, Karger, 2010, vol 28, pp 120–127

Methodological Problems in the Study of Contagious Yawning

Matthew W. Campbell · Frans B.M. de Waal

Living Links Center, Yerkes National Primate Research Center, Emory University, Atlanta, Ga., USA

Abstract

The recent interest in contagious yawning has raised several challenges as the varied methods of testing have left some unresolved issues. We do not know how differences in key variables affect the observed rates of yawning, and we highlight these as being in need of direct testing. Different researchers analyze their results differently, and we make some recommendations for more rigorous, thorough and informative analyses. Ultimately, problems arise when authors compare studies that used different methods and different analyses without acknowledging how these differences may have affected the results. In these cases, authors make inappropriate comparisons, which lead to conclusions that add confusion to the literature. Our goal in raising awareness of these issues is to generate new experiments and improve the discussion of existing research. With its link to empathy, a more standardized study of contagious yawning may be a useful tool for a variety of disciplines.

Recently there has been renewed interest in the study of contagious yawning. More research on contagious yawning has been published in the span of 2000–2009 than in the previous 2 decades (and even longer) combined. The cause of this renewed interest is the theoretical link between contagious yawning and empathy [1, 2], which has been supported empirically [3, 4]. Since the early experiments on contagious yawning [5–8], the study of this phenomenon has employed developmental [9], comparative [10–14], neurological [15–18] and mental health [19–21] approaches in a pursuit that is beginning to formulate a varied body of research. However, the now numerous studies employed different methods of experimentation and analysis with different strengths and weaknesses, which complicates efforts to compare results across studies. Focusing on experimental manipulations of contagious yawning, which have been far more numerous than naturalistic observations [4], our goal of this chapter is to discuss some of these problems, propose some solutions, and highlight some unanswered questions to facilitate future experiments and discourse.

Problems in Experimental Design

When trying to compare results across studies, the first challenge is the different ways people test contagious yawning. The most fundamental aspects of design, what is presented and how, vary so much that no two studies by different sets of authors have employed the same methods (table 1).

Three variables in particular differ more frequently than others:

(1) The duration of the yawn shown ranges from 3 to 9 s (table 1), with some studies not reporting this detail. This magnitude of difference is small, and there is ambiguity in the length of the actual yawn within the stated length of a clip (i.e. how much neutral-expression lead-time and lag-time there was). As all researchers were attempting to show more or less 'typical' yawns, relatively small differences in duration may not influence the results greatly. Nonetheless, no one has expressly studied whether the duration of a stimulus yawn influences rates of contagion.

(2) Much more challenging is that the number of yawns displayed to the subjects ranges from 1 to 140. Of the 18 studies that presented yawns, there are 13 different total number of yawns shown. This is an enormous magnitude of variation, with the added wrinkle that in some experiments all of the clips were shown in 1 session, whereas in others they were shown in multiple sessions. We do not know if the number of yawns viewed by the subjects influences the rate of contagion. Does watching more yawns induce more individuals to yawn? Does watching more yawns induce more yawns from the same individuals? The obvious co-variable that may also contribute to yawning rates is the amount of time that the subjects are observed. The longer subjects are observed, the more likely one will observe yawning. These variables, time and the number of yawns presented, can be manipulated independently, and this awaits testing. In the meantime, we need to be cautious when comparing relative rates of contagious yawning between studies with even moderately different durations of exposure. Many studies make these comparisons without acknowledging that the methods differ in potentially important ways.

(3) Another critical aspect of design is the control. There is no consensus about what makes for the ideal control. Studies have used smiles, coughs, laughs, mouths opening and closing (also called gaping), still faces and species-specific expressions (for 3 comparative studies). The merits of different controls may be argued. Some may support gaping as it mimics much of the motor pattern of a yawn, yet is a meaningless expression (note: Nahab et al. [17] had a reason to use this expression specific to using fMRI). Conversely, it can be argued that gaping does not include, and therefore control for, motor activity in the eye region the way smiles, laughs and species-specific expressions do, which Provine [7] demonstrated was important for the perception of yawns. Since there has been no comparison of yawn rates in response to these different expressions, we have no data on whether any are better or worse controls than the others. However, significant differences in yawning rates when comparing yawns and controls have been detected using all of these expressions except coughs

Table 1. Studies on yawning

First author and reference	Subjects	Control expression	Duration of yawn clip	Number of expo-sures	Apparatus size
Anderson [9]	87 children (3–11 years old)	smile	unreported	17	unreported
Anderson [10]	6 adult chimpanzees	open mouth movements	unreported	40	35-cm monitor
Arnott [18]	10 adult humans	breath, scrambled yawn (auditory)	mean ± SD: 6 ± 1.16 s	40	NA, auditory only
Baenninger [8]	40 adult humans	none	unreported for video and live presentation	1? unclear	live presentation, and unreported for video
Campbell [14]	24 adult chimpanzees	play face, hoot, tooth clack	9 s	90	48-cm monitor
Giganti [21]	children: 7 high-functioning ASD, 10 low-functioning ASD, 10 TD	smile	5 s	20	unreported
Harr [13]	15 juvenile and adult dogs	gape	3–5s	10	unreported
Joly-Mascheroni [12]	29 adult dogs	gape	live presentation	10–19	live presentation
Moore [5]	36 adult humans	none	live presentation	5	unreported
Nahab [17]	18 adult humans	gape, cough, no movement	4 s	20	unreported
Paukner [11]	22 stumptail macaques (18 adult, 3 sub-adult, 1 infant)	open mouth movements	4.5 s	140	43-cm monitor
Platek [3]	65 adult humans	laughing	7 s	8	12.1 × 10 cm window on a monitor
Platek [15]	10 adult humans	laughing	7 s	15	fMRI goggles
Provine [6]	66 adult humans	smile	5 s	30	53-cm monitor
Provine [7]	360 adult humans	smile	5 s	30	43-cm monitor
Schurmann [16]	30 adult humans	mouth and tongue movement	24–27 s for 2 clips	6? unclear	unreported
Senju [19]	children: 24 ASD, 25 TD	gape	7 s	6	30.5-cm monitor
Senju [20]	children: 31 ASD, 31 TD	gape	7 s	6	30.5-cm monitor

The 4 studies with numerous NA entries are the 4 fMRI studies that could not observe actual yawns from the subjects due to the restrictions on head movement necessary for brain imaging. TD = Typical developers.

Post-exposure observation (for build-up effect)	Yawn recording method	Asked about feeling like yawning	Yawn vs. control comparison, Population-level	Yawn vs. control comparison, Individual-level
5 min	experimenter in room	Yes	Not tested	Not tested
3 min	videotaped	Nonhuman subjects	*t*-test, NS	binomial, 2 of 6 subjects significant
NA	NA	Yes	NA	NA
none	experimenter in room	Yes	Not tested	Not tested
5 min	videotaped	Nonhuman subjects	*t*-test, $p = 0.003$	binomial, 6 of 23 subjects significant
none	videotaped	No	Wilcoxon, $p = 0.01$	Not tested
3 min	experimenter in room	Nonhuman subjects	*t*-test, NS	binomial, 1 of 15 subjects significant
5 min	experimenter in room and videotaped	Nonhuman subjects	McNemar, $p < 0.001$	Not tested
none	experimenter in room and recorded by subject	Yes	Not tested	Not tested
NA	NA	Yes	NA	NA
3 min	experimenter out of room	Nonhuman subjects	Wilcoxon, $p = 0.02$	Not tested (but some appear significant on the graph)
none	experimenter out of room	No	Not tested (a significant Wilcoxon can be inferred from the results)	Not tested
NA	NA	No	NA	NA
none	recorded by subject	No	Chi-square, $p < 0.01$	Not tested
none	recorded by subject	No	Chi-square, $p < 0.02$	Not tested
NA	NA	Yes	NA	NA
1 min	videotaped	No	Wilcoxon, $p = 0.038$ (TD condition only)	Not tested
1 min	videotaped	No	Wilcoxon, NS	Not tested

and still faces, which have only been used once in an fMRI study [17]. Therefore, the specific control expression selected may not be important, as multiple expressions seem to turn up baseline levels of yawning. It would be interesting to know if yawning rates in response to any of these expressions differ from watching a neutral face, or even a blank screen. When selecting a control, it stands to reason that one should not use an extremely arousing expression, such as fear, but we reiterate that there has been no research comparing yawning rates to different controls.

There are many more methodological details that differ between studies, as can be seen in table 1, and the same comment applies: these details have not been studied for their effect on contagious yawning. We chose to highlight 3 aspects of methodology that we feel have the biggest potential to impact rates of contagion. The duration of the yawn clip may not be important, ultimately, and many different control expressions may do an equally good job of eliciting a baseline rate of yawning. However, the number of the yawn clips shown, with the co-variable of the amount of time the subjects are observed, has the potential to drastically impact the results and therefore interpretation. Research in this area is gravely needed, both for future experiments, and to more accurately compare existing studies that vary greatly in this domain.

Problems in Analysis

What qualifies as yawn contagion? This simple question has no clear answer in the literature. Whereas all authors agree on what yawn contagion is: a yawn stimulated by another yawn, there is no agreement on how to measure it. The most common analytical methods assess population-level differences between yawn and control conditions using either parametric (e.g. Student's t test) or non-parametric (e.g. Wilcoxon signed-rank test, χ^2, McNemar's test) statistics. Buried within the parametric or non-parametric distinction is a subtle difference in what these tests measure. The t test and Wilcoxon examine whether there were more *yawns* in the yawn condition than the control; χ^2 and the McNemar variant examine whether more *subjects* yawned in the yawn than the control condition, regardless of the magnitude of response. The χ^2 and McNemar may be of more limited use as they require a lot of 0's in the control condition. Whether one type of test is preferable to the other is not clear, but experimenters and readers need to be aware of the differences.

While relatively rare, a few studies did not do a statistical test between their yawn and control responses, which is a significant oversight. Population-level tests tell us whether one group as a whole is different from another, but they do not inform us about any one individual. Less commonly used, a few studies (curiously, all studies of non-human animals) have also employed individual-level statistics in the form of binomials. Binomials compare one individual's rate of response between two conditions. This test can identify individuals who show a strong difference in yawning regardless of the population-level statistics. In short, they can identify high-performers. The limitation to binomials is that they are not sensitive to small differences that may be meaningful and consistent within a population, hence the need for population-level statistics. These two levels of analysis should be seen as complementary: population-level tests tell us whether one group as a group differs from another, whereas individual-level tests identify particularly strong performers within a population. One is not better than the other; rather, they test different questions. All experimental manipulations of contagious yawning should compare the response to the yawn stimulus to the control stimulus. This is mandatory. Our suggestion is that a thorough analysis should contain statistics at both population and individual levels.

One particular result that is frequently reported but difficult to interpret is the percent of subjects showing contagious yawning. The difficulty arises because first one must define operationally what qualifies a subject as showing contagious yawning. An operational definition of contagious yawning has not been made explicit in any study reporting this result. There are at least 3 different ways one could operationally define whether a subject shows contagious yawning: (1) if subject A yawns at all during the yawn condition, regardless of how many times or if the subjects yawns at all, or even more frequently, during the control; (2) if subject A yawns more in the yawn condition than the control; (3) if subject A yawns significantly more during the yawn than the control on a binomial test. Method 1 is the most liberal (and most commonly used), and method 3 is the most conservative. Using our own data on chimpanzees as an example [14], these three different methods yield percentages of contagiously yawning subjects of 65, 56.5 and 26%, respectively. Thus, when authors compare percentages calculated with different methods [calculation method not reported in: 10, 12, 13, 21] they end up drawing conclusions from heterogeneous comparisons.

Secondly, how many individuals are observed to yawn during the yawn condition will depend to some extent upon the duration of the experiment. The longer a subject is observed, the more likely one will see a yawn. This is not a problem when comparing results within a study since the yawn and control conditions will be the same, but when comparing results between studies, there are serious problems if one study watched subjects for 5 min, and another for 20 min. Comparing yawns per minute, as opposed to the absolute number of yawning individuals, is one way to control for this.

The last problem we raise with this comparison is that a population that naturally yawns at high rates will look like possessing more contagion when compared to a population that naturally yawns very little, regardless of how these populations perform between yawn and control conditions. One can imagine a population that yawns a lot spontaneously, with no significant difference between the yawn and the control condition, and another population that yawns very little, but does show a significant difference. Would it be accurate to conclude that the first population shows more contagious yawning than the second? It is the difference between the yawn and control conditions that indicates susceptibility to contagion. A better comparison would be to look at the magnitudes of the difference in response between yawn and control conditions. Therefore, we would look at which populations show strongly significant differences, moderately significant differences, or no differences at all. This allows each population to control for itself and its own natural rates of yawning, as well as controlling for different methodologies, as discussed above.

Conclusions

Our analysis yields the following broad recommendations:

- new controlled experiments on variables of methodology, specifically how the number of yawns shown, the time duration of the experiment, and different control expressions affect rates of yawning;
- demonstrating yawn contagion experimentally requires a statistically significant difference between the response to a yawn stimulus and a control;
- calculations of percent of subjects showing yawn contagion are not informative;
- when making comparisons between different studies, authors must acknowledge how different methods and analyses may influence the results.

The last 10 years has seen a resurgence in interest in contagious yawning. We are very excited about the varied directions research has taken, and we hope these trends continue. Studying key variables of presenting yawns will be beneficial for two reasons: (1) it will facilitate comparisons across studies, including clarifying which variables in past studies may be important; (2) it will bring us closer to a standardized methodology, which may be useful as a diagnostic test for some mental health conditions [3, 19–21]. Answering these basic questions and limiting confusion in the literature will facilitate using contagious yawning as a serious tool to better understand how empathy functions from developmental, comparative, neurological and mental health perspectives.

References

1 Lehmann HE: Yawning: a homeostatic reflex and its psychological significance. Bull Menninger Clin 1979;4:123–136.

2 Preston SD, de Waal FBM: Empathy: its ultimate and proximate bases. Behav Brain Sci 2002;25:1–72.

3 Platek SM, Critton SR, Myers TE, Gallup GG: Contagious yawning: the role of self-awareness and mental state attribution. Brain Res Cogn Brain Res 2003;17:223–227.

4 Palagi E, Leone A, Mancini G, Ferrari PF: Contagious yawning in gelada baboons as a possible expression of empathy. Proc Natl Acad Sci USA 2009;108:19262–19267.

5 Moore JE: Some psychological aspects of yawning. J Gen Psychol 1942;27:289–294.

6 Provine RR: Yawning as a stereotyped action pattern and releasing stimulus. Ethology 1986;72:109–122.

7 Provine RR: Faces as releasers of contagious yawning: an approach to face detection using normal humans subjects. Bull Psychon Soc 1989;27:211–214.

8 Baenninger R: Some comparative aspects of yawning in *Betta splendens, Homo sapiens, Panthera leo,* and *Papio sphinx.* J Comp Psychol 1987;101:349–354.

9 Anderson JR, Meno P: Psychological influences on yawning in children. Curr Psychol Lett 2003;11:1–7.

10 Anderson JR, Myowa-Yamakoshi M, Matsuzawa T: Contagious yawning in chimpanzees. Proc R Soc Lond B Biol Sci 2004;271(suppl):S468–S470.
11 Paukner A, Anderson JR: Video-induced yawning in stumptail macaques (*Macaca arctoides*). Biol Lett 2006;2:36–38.
12 Joly-Mascheroni RM, Senju A, Shepherd AJ: Dogs catch human yawns. Biol Lett 2008;4:446–448.
13 Harr AL, Gilbert VR, Philips KA: Do dogs (*Canis familiaris*) show contagious yawning? Anim Cogn 2009;12:833–837.
14 Campbell MW, Carter JD, Proctor D, Eisenberg ML, de Waal FBM: Computer animations stimulate contagious yawning in chimpanzees. Proc R Soc Lond B Biol Sci 2009;276:4255–4259.
15 Platek SM, Mohamed FB, Gallup JGG: Contagious yawning and the brain. Brain Res Cogn Brain Res 2005;23:448–452.
16 Schurmann M Hesse MD, Stephan KE, Saarela M, Zilles K, Hari R, Fink GR: Yearning to yawn: the neural basis of contagious yawning. Neuroimage 2005;24:1260–1264.
17 Nahab FB, Hattori N, Saad ZS, Hallett M: Contagious yawning and the frontal lobe: an fMRI study. Hum Brain Mapp 2009;30:1744–1751.
18 Arnott SR, Singhal A, Goodale MA: An investigation of auditory contagious yawning. Cogn Affect Behav Neurosci 2009;9:335–342.
19 Senju A, Maeda M, Kikuchi Y, Hasegawa T, Tojo Y, Osanai H: Absence of contagious yawning in children with autism spectrum disorder. Biol Lett 2007; 3:706–708.
20 Senju A, Kikuchi Y, Akechi H, Hasegawa T, Tojo Y, Osanai H: Brief report: does eye contact induce contagious yawning in children with autism spectrum disorder? J Autism Dev Disord 2009;39:1598–1602.
21 Giganti F, Esposito Ziello M: Contagious and spontaneous yawning in autistic and typically developing children. Curr Psychol Lett 2009;25:1–11.

Matthew W. Campbell
Living Links Center, Yerkes National Primate Research Center, Emory University
Atlanta, GA 30072 (USA)
Tel. +1 404 727 9071, Fax +1 404 727 9069
E-Mail matthew.campbell@emory.edu

Walusinski O (ed): The Mystery of Yawning in Physiology and Disease.
Front Neurol Neurosci. Basel, Karger, 2010, vol 28, pp 128–133

Exploring Yawning with Neuroimaging

Fatta B. Nahab

University of Miami Miller School of Medicine, Miami, Fla., USA

Abstract

The neural mechanisms responsible for spontaneous yawning as well as contagious yawning are not well characterized. Neuroimaging is an essential tool for helping to identify the seminal neural structures and their inter-related functions to carry out this complex stereotyped motor program. Studies to date have explored the structural neural correlates of yawning through a series of lesion-based case reports and identified participatory structures at various levels of the central nervous system. Functional neuroimaging methods like fMRI have also shed led on the genesis of contagious yawning, though cohesive models explaining the neural mechanisms of contagious motor programs such as yawning remain limited.

The genesis and function of the yawn has baffled humans since ancient times. Yawning requires no conscious motor planning and manifests in a stereotypic manner regardless of the animal involved, human or otherwise. This primitive motor program requires the concerted activity of facial, oral, laryngeal, pharyngeal, thoracic and abdominal musculature. Despite the ubiquity of spontaneous yawning across species, only primates [1] and possibly dogs [2, 3] yawn to a contagion, or in response to viewing, hearing or simply thinking about a yawn [4].

Physiology of Yawning

Despite numerous theories regarding the mechanism or function of yawning, little is known about the underlying physiological mechanisms of this primitive behavior. Attempts to isolate the neural correlates of yawning have yielded a wide range of results. Involvement of the brainstem cranial nuclei is clear, since these neural structures mediate the outflow to the muscles required to carry out a yawn. Seizures involving the brainstem have been associated with abnormal behaviors including head bobbing, sniffing and yawning [5]. The upstream mechanisms that trigger spontaneous yawning or the brain regions involved in the processing of contagious yawning remain poorly understood.

Various studies have, however, shed light on the neural structures involved in yawning. A report by Jurko and Andy [6] observed yawning during hyperventilation that occurred in certain patients who underwent thalamotomy. All of the lesions that elicited yawning (during the routine recording of electroencephalograms) were localized to the medial portion of the centro-median nucleus of the thalamus. In rats, electrical and chemical stimulation of the paraventricular nucleus (PVN) of the hypothalamus also stimulated yawning [7, 8]. Microinjection of histamine into the medial parvocellular subdivision of the PVN also elicited yawns and an arousal shift was observed using electrocorticography, as evidenced by lower voltage and faster rhythms. Microinjection of HTMT (histamine trifluoromethyl toluidide) dimaleate, a histamine H_1 receptor agonist, into the PVN also caused the yawning/arousal response, whereas pretreatment with pyrilamine, an H_1 receptor antagonist, inhibited the histamine-induced yawning behavior [9].

Neuroimaging of Yawning

The advent of high-resolution structural and functional neuroimaging modalities such as MRI and PET provide new and more sensitive methods to explore the neural underpinnings of yawning. Lesion-based inferences utilizing structural imaging have identified additional components of the larger yawn neural network. Walusinski et al. [10] reported that in some cases of hemiplegia following a stroke in the internal capsule, yawning was associated with the involuntary raising of the subject's paralyzed arm. Two additional cases of brainstem strokes involving the upper pons and the ponto-mesencephalic junction also presented with transient excessive pathological yawning [11].

Despite the large number of brain regions implicated in spontaneous yawning, little has been ascertained about how these regions interact as a cohesive network to generate a yawn. Newer neuroimaging methods such as blood-oxygen-level-dependent functional MRI (BOLD-fMRI) provide this ability to characterize the neural network. fMRI may also utilize behavioral paradigms to probe the mechanisms underlying contagious yawning. Schurmann et al. [12] utilized BOLD-fMRI to explore the neural correlates of the yawn contagion, and hypothesized that yawning would not significantly activate mirror neuron networks since yawns are produced automatically without the need for imitation. The investigators conducted a block-design experiment whereby participants viewed videos of unknown actors performing yawns or control movements involving the tongue for approximately 25 s, interspersed by periods of rest. Their findings showed differences between yawn and control stimuli in the right posterior superior temporal sulcus (STS) and bilaterally in the anterior STS. In addition, they identified no yawn-specific activations in Broca's area that supported their hypothesis, suggesting the mirror neuron system (MNS) was not involved in the genesis of yawning to a contagion. Finally, they noted that their subjects' yawn susceptibility negatively covaried with amygdalar BOLD activity and suggested this was related to 'the effectiveness of yawn contagion and the face-processing-related emotional analysis during social interaction'.

To expand on prior work demonstrating that susceptibility to contagious yawning was negatively correlated with schizotypal personality traits, Platek et al. [13] conducted an fMRI study to investigate whether theory of mind or empathy networks were activated while subjects viewed yawn videos [14]. This study involved 10 subjects undergoing fMRI while viewing 7-second videos consisting of 1 of 3 conditions: neutral, laughing and yawning. The findings provided evidence for the hypothesis that contagious yawning may be a primitive form of empathic modeling based on the activation of the posterior cingulate and precuneus. Additional activations in the bilateral thalami and parahippocampal gyri were attributed to visual and sensory processing of the stimuli. It should be noted that a more recent fMRI study exploring the neural correlates of hearing a yawn did demonstrate involvement of the MNS [15].

Based on these preliminary findings, our own group hoped to unify and expand on the previous findings regarding the yawn neural network by exploring the brain responses induced when subjects viewed yawns and similar non-contagious facial actions [16]. We used single video clips of 4 seconds' duration showing an unfamiliar actor performing 1 of 4 facial expressions: yawning, gaping, coughing and a "blank" expressionless face with limited blinking. We used a single stimulus set to avoid confounds related to viewing novel faces or facial expressions. The blank face and cough stimuli served to control for facial perception and visual motion, whereas the gape action involved the actor opening the mouth wide then closing with similar timing to a yawn, but while maintaining the eyes wide open and having a more robotic appearance. Thus gaping mimicked all aspects of facial movement, complexity and timing associated with yawning, without conveying the behavioral or emotional components of yawning. To obtain a more objective measure of the various stimuli, we measured the relative motion characteristics over time (MoCharT) using an inhouse [Matsuhashi M, unpublished] Matlab script (Mathworks) that compared frame-by-frame pixel changes as an approximation of overall motion (fig. 1).

The shorter stimulus duration and slow event-related design we implemented allowed for the display of a complete yawn cycle, while minimizing potential confounders such as response habituation or potentiation. Eighteen healthy right-handed subjects participated, while remaining naïve to the experimental goals. At the completion of the MRI session, subjects were informed about the goals of the experiment and completed a binary questionnaire describing their susceptibility to contagious yawning, both in general and during the experiment.

Our fMRI results provided both expected and novel results. In addition to standard activations in visual (all stimuli) and visual motion areas (cough, gape,

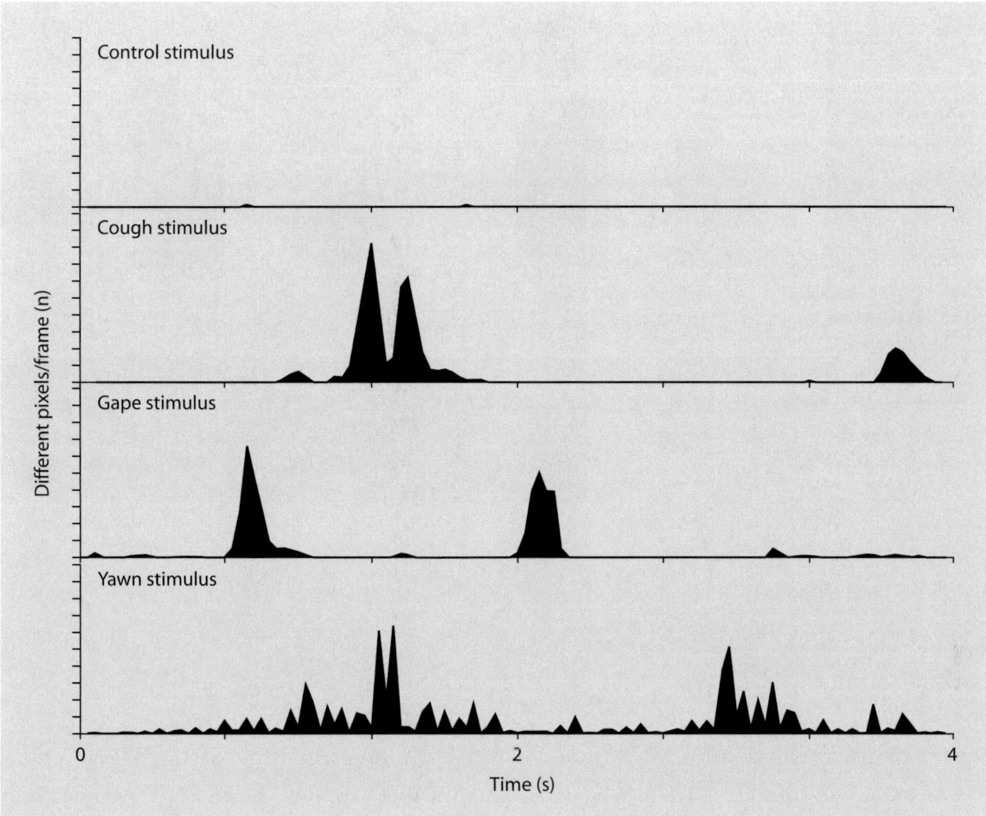

Fig. 1. Relative visual motion characteristics over time (MoCharT) of our 4 stimulus classes.

yawn stimuli), we found common activations in right inferior frontal cortex and right STS during the cough and gape stimuli. The gape condition showed a number of additional activations, including the bilateral ventral premotor areas, the parahippocampal gyrus near the ventral posterior cingulate (BA 23) and pre-supplementary motor area. For our contrast of interest (yawn-gape), we found a significant difference only in the region of the ventromedial prefrontal cortex (vmPFC; fig. 2).

The findings of activations in inferior frontal cortex, STS, ventral premotor and the posterior cingulate validated prior study results while demonstrating their association with our non-contagious control stimuli. Despite the activation of human mirror neuron areas, such as the inferior frontal cortex and STS, we found no significant MNS activations in our yawn-gape contrast since these regions were involved in both conditions and unlikely to be the primary regions mediating contagious motor programs such as yawning. The novel finding of vmPFC activation associated with viewing contagious yawning does however seem a reasonable candidate

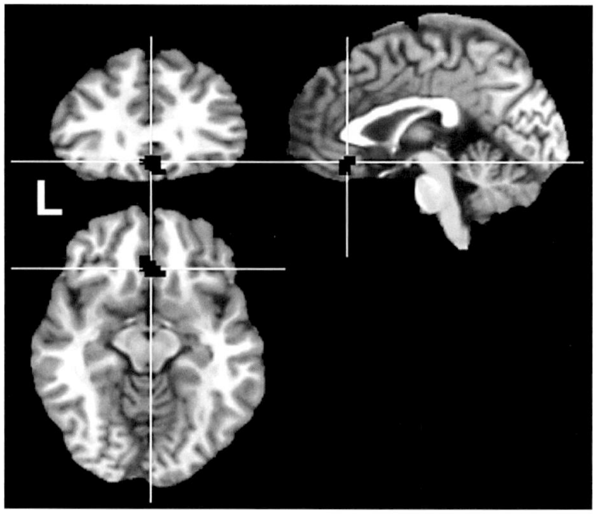

Fig. 2. Results of yawn vs. gape contrast showing significant ($p = 0.05$, corrected) activation in the ventromedial prefrontal cortex (local cluster maximum center of mass in Talairach coordinates at $x = 1.5$, $y = 25.5$, $z = -9.5$; $Z_{max} = 3.95$).

region. The vmPFC has been associated with emotional processing of internal and external stimuli and representation of emotional responses [17]. The identification of a cortical correlate of contagious yawning may seem unlikely, considering its primitive origins and its association with previously reported lower brain regions such as the hypothalamus and brainstem. A cortical 'releasing' mechanism, however, helps to explain why yawning is ubiquitous while contagious yawning is primarily restricted to humans and non-human primates. Furthermore, the role of the vmPFC in contagious yawning may explain the findings of Anderson and Meno [18] showing that contagious yawning did not develop in children below the age of 5 years. We hypothesize that the processing of contagious motor programs only begin after the child has reached some developmental or biological milestone (e.g. axonal myelination, synaptic plasticity or empathic processing), and that this process may be heralded by the disappearance of other primitive reflexes in the toddler.

Summary

The neural structures involved in the generation of the yawn appear to span multiple levels of the neural axis, including the brainstem, subcortical regions and prefrontal cortex. The roles and interplay of these regions in the motor production of the yawn, as well as the processing of contagious yawning, remain poorly understood. Further work is needed to integrate our knowledge of contagious motor programs such as yawning into a model explaining the functional roles of each brain region and its contribution to the larger neural network.

References

1 Anderson JR, Myowa-Yamakoshi M, Matsuzawa T: Contagious yawning in chimpanzees. Proc Biol Sci 2004;271:S468–S470.

2 Joly-Mascheroni RM, Senju A, Shepherd AJ: Dogs catch human yawns. Biol Lett 2008;4:446–448.

3 Harr AL, Gilbert VR, Phillips KA: Do dogs (*Canis familiaris*) show contagious yawning? Anim Cogn 2009;12:833–837.

4 Provine RR: Yawning. Am Sci 2005;93:532–539.

5 Qian XB, Andy OJ, Dearman C, Andrews M, Rockhold RW: Cocaine-induced brainstem seizures and behavior. Integr Physiol Behav Sci 1992;27:117–129.

6 Jurko MF, Andy OJ: Post-lesion yawning and thalamotomy site. Appl Neurophysiol 1975;38:73–79.

7 Sato-Suzuki I, Kita I, Oguri M, Arita H: Stereotyped yawning responses induced by electrical and chemical stimulation of paraventricular nucleus of the rat. J Neurophysiol 1998;80:2765–2775.

8 Kita I, Kubota N, Yanagita S, Motoki C: Intracerebroventricular administration of corticotropin-releasing factor antagonist attenuates arousal response accompanied by yawning behavior in rats. Neurosci Lett 2008;433:205–208.

9 Seki Y, Sato-Suzuki I, Kita I, Oguri M, Arita H: Yawning/cortical activation induced by microinjection of histamine into the paraventricular nucleus of the rat. Behav Brain Res 2002;134:75–82.

10 Walusinski O, Quoirin E, Neau JP: Parakinesia brachialis oscitans (in French). Rev Neurol (Paris) 2005;161:193–200.

11 Cattaneo L, Cucurachi L, Chierici E, Pavesi G: Pathological yawning as a presenting symptom of brain stem ischaemia in two patients. J Neurol Neurosurg Psychiatry 2006;77:98–100.

12 Schurmann M, Hesse MD, Stephan KE, Saarela M, Zilles K, Hari R, et al: Yearning to yawn: the neural basis of contagious yawning. Neuroimage 2005;24:1260–1264.

13 Platek SM, Critton SR, Myers TE, Gallup GG: Contagious yawning: the role of self-awareness and mental state attribution. Brain Res Cogn Brain Res 2003;17:223–227.

14 Platek SM, Mohamed FB, Gallup GG Jr: Contagious yawning and the brain. Brain Res Cogn Brain Res 2005;23:448–452.

15 Arnott SR, Singhal A, Goodale MA: An investigation of auditory contagious yawning. Cogn Affect Behav Neurosci 2009;9:335–342.

16 Nahab FB, Hattori N, Saad ZS, Hallett M: Contagious yawning and the frontal lobe: an fMRI study. Hum Brain Mapp 2009;30:1744–1751.

17 Bush G, Luu P, Posner MI: Cognitive and emotional influences in anterior cingulate cortex. Trends Cogn Sci 2000;4:215–222.

18 Anderson JR, Meno P: Psychological influences on yawning in children. Curr Psychol Lett 2006;2:11.

Asst. Prof. Fatta B. Nahab, MD
University of Miami Miller School of Medicine
1120 NW 14th Street, Suite 1347 (C215)
Miami, FL 33136 (USA)
Tel. +1 305 243 4075, Fax +1 305 243 7081, E-Mail FNahab@med.miami.edu

Walusinski O (ed): The Mystery of Yawning in Physiology and Disease.
Front Neurol Neurosci. Basel, Karger, 2010, vol 28, pp 134–139

Associated Movements in Hemiplegic Limbs during Yawning

Ramachandran Meenakshisundaram[a] · Ponniah Thirumalaikolundusubramanian[b] · Olivier Walusinski[d] · Arunachalam Muthusundari[c] · Shah Sweni[e]

[a]Madras Medical College, Chennai, [b]Chennai Medical College Hospital & Research Center, Trichy, [c]Tirunelveli Medical College, Tirunelveli, India; [d]General Practice, Brou, France; [e]University of Debrecen, Medical and Health Science Center, Debrecen, Hungary

Abstract

Background: Yawning is phylogenetically ancient and associated with a stereotyped behavioral pattern. **Objective:** To describe the pattern of associated movements observed in hemiplegic limbs during yawning and its relationship to gender, laterality of hemiplegia and muscle tone. **Material and Methods:** An observational study was designed for 75 patients with newly detected anterior circulatory stroke due to ischemia or hemorrhage in the internal capsule region. The subjects were free from any arthropathy, autoimmune disease, muscular disorders and injury/deformity. **Results:** There were 48 males and 27 females, whose median ages were 48 and 47 years, respectively. The median yawning onset times after stroke in males and females were 36 and 38 h, respectively. Associated movements in hemiplegic limbs during yawning were minimal and observed in 59 hemiplegics (78.6%); significantly more were seen in males (83%) vs. females (70%), left-sided (94%) vs. right-sided hemiplegics (64%), those with hypotonia (87%) vs. hypertonia (61%), and in the upper limbs (91%) vs. lower limbs (83%) and proximal (72%) vs. distal joints (29%), irrespective of limb. **Conclusion:** The appearance of associated movements in hemiplegic limbs indicates the return of ancestral function observed in quadrupeds. However, further studies are needed to ascertain the reasons for such variations and determine how to utilize these movements in rehabilitation programs.

Yawning is a phylogenetically old stereotyped phenomena. A yawn is a paroxysmal cycle characterized by a standard cascade of movements over 5- to 10-second periods, and the pattern is often repetitive. Associated movements in hemiplegic limbs during yawning have rarely been discussed in lecture classes and seldom looked for during clinical rounds. Historically, in the year 1794, Erasmus Darwin [1] was the first to describe movements of a paralyzed arm in hemiplegic limbs which were completely disobedient to the will. John Abercrombie [2] described the same, with the movements followed by a reduction in paralysis.

The clinical phenomenon of involuntary movements of paralyzed upper limbs in hemiplegics during yawning was coined as 'parakinesia brachialis oscitans' [3]. The reports describing associated movements in hemiplegic limbs during yawning are scarce, and many described upper rather than lower limb movements. Therefore, the present study was undertaken to find out the associated movements in hemiplegic limbs during yawning and their relationship with hemiplegia, muscle tone and gender.

Material and Methods

An observational study was designed to find out the associated movements in hemiplegic limbs after institutional ethical clearance and informed consent. A total of 75 cases of newly diagnosed acute-onset anterior territory stroke due to ischemia or hemorrhage (as evidenced by brain CT) with lesions in the internal capsule were considered. These cases were free from any arthropathy, autoimmune disorders, muscular diseases, or injury/deformity in the limbs. Two of the family members (caregivers) who were looking after the patients were taught and trained to observe the movements of the hemiplegic limbs during yawning by video clips and personal coaching. Then, caregivers were asked to demonstrate the movements they observed in the patient using their limbs while remaining lying. The degree of movement was gauged on a 3-point scale as described by Mulley [4]: no, minimal or considerable movement. Only those who were able to understand the requirements and reproduce the movements were considered for the study.

The clinical details and laboratory investigations were recorded. Neurological status was assessed using the NIH Stroke Scale [5]. These cases were followed up in the hospital during first 7 days. Data were analyzed by simple descriptive statistics and McNemar's test for correlated proportions [6].

Results

There were 48 males and 27 females; their median ages were 48 (27–81) and 47 (36–70) years, respectively. All of them were right-handed. Among the cases, 39 presented with right-sided hemiplegia, 36 with left-sided hemiplegia, 52 with hypotonia and 23 with hypertonia. The time taken to develop the first yawning episode in hemiplegics varied from 12 to 86 h in males and 11 to 70 h in females, with medians of 36 and 38 h, respectively. Associated movements in the hemiplegic limbs were noticed in 78.6% of the cases. These were present more often in males (83%) than in females (70%), and the difference was significant statistically ($p < 0.05$). Among males and females (respectively), associated movements of both upper and lower limbs on the hemiplegic side during yawning were observed in 32 and 12 cases, the upper limbs alone in 7 and 3 cases, and the lower limbs alone in 1 and 4 cases. However, the occurrence of movements of hemiplegic limbs during yawning was independent of the upper and lower limbs.

Associated movements were noticed in 45 hypotonic (87%) and 14 hypertonic (61%) hemiplegic patients, and the difference was significant statistically ($p < 0.01$).

Table 1. Pattern of movements in hemiplegic limbs during yawning

	Males (n = 40)			Females (n = 19)			Males and females		Grand total (n = 59)
	right	left	total	right	left	total	right	left	
Shoulder									
Abduction	9	8	17	4	4	8	13	12	25
Flexion	8	8	16	4	1	5	12	9	21
Extension	1	4	5	–	1	1	1	5	6
Elbow									
Flexion	3	3	6	3	–	3	6	3	9
Extension	–	1	1	–	–	–	–	1	1
Hand (Wrist)									
Extension	–	2	2	–	–	–	–	2	2
Flexion	–	1	1	1	–	1	1	1	2
Closing finger	–	–	–	–	2	2	–	2	2
Stretching finger	–	–	–	–	2	2	–	2	2
Hip									
Flexion	8	9	17	5	3	8	13	12	25
Extension	1	–	1	–	–	–	1	–	1
Abduction	–	–	–	–	2	2	–	2	2
External rotation	–	2	2	2	–	2	2	2	4
Internal rotation	–	1	1	–	–	–	–	1	1
Knee									
Flexion	2	3	5	3	1	4	5	4	9
Ankle									
Plantar flexion	1	3	4	–	–	–	1	3	4

Also, associated movements observed in 34 left-sided (94%) and 25 right-sided (64%) hemiplegics, although this was not significant. The pattern of movements observed in hemiplegic limbs in relation to gender and laterality of hemiplegia is depicted in table 1. Patterns of associated movements observed among patients with one or other movement (n = 59) were: abduction, flexion and extension in the shoulder among 42, 36 and 10%, respectively; flexion and extension of the elbow in 15 and 1.6%, respectively; flexion and extension of the wrist in 3.3% each; closing and stretching of the fingers in 3.3% each. Similarly associated movements observed in the hip of hemiplegic side were flexion, external rotation, abduction, extension and internal rotation (42, 7, 3.3, 1.6 and 1.6% respectively). Flexion of the knee was seen in 15.3% and plantar flexion of the ankle in 6.7%. In our group, movement in the proximal joints alone was seen in 33 cases, distal joints alone in 7 cases, and both in 10 cases.

Table 2. Statistical association of the factors among hemiplegic patients with movements associated to yawning

	2-tailed p value	OR	95% CI
Males (40) vs. females (19)	0.0086*	2.11	1.22–3.63
Isolated upper (10) vs. lower limbs (5)	0.3017	2.00	0.68–5.85
Left- (34) vs. right-sided hemiplegia (25)	0.2975	1.36	0.81–2.28
Hypotonia (45) vs. hypertonia (14)	0.00006*	3.21	1.76–5.86
Isolated proximal (33) vs. distal joints (7)	0.00004*	4.71	2.09–10.66

Figures in parentheses refer to the number of cases. * $p \leq 0.01$.

Proximal joints include the shoulder and hip; joints distal to these were considered distal joints. There was no significant difference with regard to movement at the shoulder and hip joints. The movements were far less distal, and the difference was significant statistically ($p < 0.001$). The details of the statistical analysis are provided in table 2.

Discussion

Yawning has become a subject of interest to physiologists, pharmacologists, neurologists, psychologists and biologists, and their contributions have been recently reviewed [7]. As a result, many observations, theories and explanations have accumulated. Only at the start of 21st century, have the neurohormonal mechanisms for yawning been established. Although a final answer has not yet been agreed upon, yawning is considered to be a marker of activity of D_3 dopamine receptors.

In the present study, associated movements in hemiplegic limbs were observed in 80% of cases, which is similar to the values reported by Mulley [4]. The patterns of movement noticed in the study were minimal, and there were no violent movements. The patterns of associated movements in hemiplegic limbs are seen at different joints and vary across different series [4, 7–10]. These variations may be related to the individual responses to stimuli or the reversal of functioning capacity of adjacent neurological structures. Interestingly, such movements are more common in proximal than distal joints. This may be due to increased muscle bulk in the proximal joints. It has been suggested that comparing the associated limb movements during yawning before and after the onset of hemiplegia in the same individual will throw more light on these variations in movement patterns.

An ischemic attack affecting the territory of lenticulostriate arteries and damaging the internal capsule leads to complete hemiplegia due to the lesion of the pyramidal tract with sparing of the extrapyramidal pathways. Automatic synchronization of the ventilatory cycle with gait is observed in quadrupeds, but not in humans due to bipedalism. After the onset of stroke, cortical control is interrupted and the adjacent neurological structures retrieve the ancestral function. Hence, during movement of the diaphragm while yawning, the paralyzed arm receives motor stimulation from the lateral reticular nucleus of medulla, which is involved in ventilation and locomotion in animals. Topper et al. [11] suggested the possibility of an emotional motor system to explain these movements in the hemiplegic limbs during yawning.

Though associated movements have been noticed in the hemiplegic limbs, doctors and physiotherapists taking care of such patients should realize that associated movement has no prognostic value [4]. Mulley [4] did not find any association between associated movements and gender or laterality of hemiplegia. In this study, movements were noticed more in males, proximal joints and those with left-sided hemiplegia and hypotonia. Further studies are warranted to find out the reasons for variation in the movements and optimal ways of utilizing these results in the rehabilitation programs.

Strength and Limitations

The strengths of our study were rigid inclusion and exclusion criteria as well as careful monitoring of movements. Interestingly, passive movements of hemiplegic limbs during sneezing, coughing and laughing were not monitored.

Acknowledgments

We would like to thank Dr. Andrew G. Dean and Mr. Erik Knudsen of the Center for Disease Control and Prevention for their guidance and help with the statistical calculations.

References

1 Darwin E: Zoonomia or the Laws of Organic Life. London, Johnson J, 1801.
2 Abercrombie J: Pathological and Practical Researches on Diseases of the Brain and the Spinal Cord. Edinburgh, Waugh and Innes, 1828.
3 Walusinski O, Quoirin E, Neau JP: Parakinesia brachialis oscitans (in French). Rev Neurol (Paris) 2005;161:193–200.
4 Mulley G: Associated reactions in the hemiplegic arm. Scand J Rehabil Med 1982;14:117–120.
5 National Institutes of Health: NIH Stroke Scale. Bethesda, NIH, 2008. www.ninds.nih.gov/doctors/NIH_Stroke_Scale_Booklet.pdf.
6 Lowry R: VassarStats interactive statistical calculations. 2008 (accessed 16 November 2009). http://faculty.vassar.edu/lowry/propcorr.html.
7 Walusinski O: Yawning in diseases. Euro Neurol 2009;62:180–187.
8 Walshe F: On the genesis and physiological significances of spasticity and other disorders of motor innervation, with a consideration of the functional relationships of the pyramidal system. Brain 1919; 42:1–28.

9 Walshe F: On certain tonic postural reflexes in hemiplegia with special reference to the so-called associated movements. Brain 1923;46:1–37.
10 Thompson H: Associated movements in hemiplegia: their origin and physiological significance. Brain 1903;26:514–523.
11 Topper R, Mull M, Nacimiento W: Involuntary stretching during yawning in patients with pyramidal tract lesions: further evidence for the existence of an independent emotional motor system. Eur J Neurol 2003;10:495–499.

Ramachandran Meenakshisundaram
69 Pasupathy Nagar
Madurai 625017 (India)
Tel. 0091 9486258115, Fax 0091 431 4298877
E-Mail rmsundar_chandran@yahoo.co.in

Walusinski O (ed): The Mystery of Yawning in Physiology and Disease.
Front Neurol Neurosci. Basel, Karger, 2010, vol 28, pp 140–155

Associated Diseases

Olivier Walusinski

General Practice, Brou, France

Abstract

Yawning is a physiological behavior and, as with all such behaviors, its deregulation is indicative of an underlying disorder. This chapter breaks this topic down into the types of yawning (incomplete, absent or excessive) and the direction of causality (triggering or relieving a disorder).

Yawning is a physiological behavior, an emotional stereotypy that indicates the homeostatic process of the mechanisms regulating rhythms – such as sleeping-waking, hunger-satiety or mating-relaxation – generated by the diencephalon. As with all physiological behaviors, its deregulation reveals disorders. However, a property unique to yawning, which is nevertheless physiological, is its ability to trigger certain disorders and, conversely, to cure others!

Can one talk about the 'disease of yawning'? Here is what H. Meige and E. Feindel wrote in 1902 in their famous book *Tics and Their Treatment* [1, p. 346]:

> Yawning and sneezing, which, like swallowing, are reflexive phenomena whose mechanism is voluntarily modified only with great difficulty, can hardly be perturbed except with respect to their frequency. Saenger (Observations on the idiopathic spasm of the tongue, *Monatsschrift für Psychiatrie und Neurologie*, January 1900, p. 77) reported on the case of a 29-year old woman who was not hysterical and who presented with episodes of yawning with rigidity in the arms, followed by rapid contractions of the tongue for around a minute. She recovered after several months. The case concerned an 'idiopathic spasm', probably some sort of tic. However, these functional anomalies of yawning or sneezing most often occur in hysterical subjects. It should also be remembered that yawning may be the aura of an epileptic seizure. Uncontrollable yawning is also seen in meningitic incidents, and in cases of tumors of the brain or cerebellum.

The analysis of clinical observations in light of the neurophysiological knowledge accumulated over a century, allows us to affirm the existence of pathological yawning, and to distinguish between its various forms: the dissatisfaction of incomplete yawning, the disappearance of yawning and the excess of repeated yawning.

Anhedonia

Frustration due to the incomplete or inharmonious development of a yawn is a frequent complaint. Yawning stretches the respiratory and facial muscles, and is sometimes associated with a generalized muscular stretching of the trunk and limbs. The yawner perceives differences in muscle tonus, a veritable and conscious extraction of the progress of the phenomenon, of its stimulus and its contextual valence, through interoceptive pathways (projections by the lateral spinothalamic tract onto the insular cortex) leading to a hedonistic perception. The dissatisfaction felt seems to be linked to an unconscious inhibition of the 'letting go' that underlies a complete yawn. Therapeutic interventions for anxiety states or for insomnia, such as relaxation or sophrology, do in fact use the control of yawning as a means of relaxation or as an anti-stress aid, a veritable proprioceptive rehabilitation of the body scheme [2, 3].

Disappearance of Yawning

Yawning is a banal action, often barely noticed or felt. It seems that its disappearance is not perceived. Complaints of missing the feeling of well-being associated with yawning, due to the absence of yawning, remain the exception. In daily life, there appear to be no particular consequences to not yawning. The reality of this fact can be questioned, since some yawns could occur without being felt or noticed. Certain extrapyramidal syndromes are accompanied by a disappearance of yawning, such as in the case of treatment with neuroleptics [4] or Parkinson's disease [5]. This disappearance indicates the activity state of the dopaminergic neurons of the paraventricular nucleus of the hypothalamus, which are necessary for yawning. Experimental pharmacology has shown the specificity of the D_3 dopamine receptors in triggering this behavior [6]. While the neuroleptics currently in use have no specific target of action, one may assume that the presence or absence of yawning in Parkinson's disease reflects the state of the neuronal population: functional or undergoing degenerative involution. The treatment of episodes of motor blocks in Parkinson's patients by apomorphine hydrochloride, a rapid-action dopaminergic stimulant, triggers yawning, as does treatment with L-DOPA, but in a less systematic fashion [7–9]. Dewey et al. [10] noted this effect in 8% of the patients they treated, and its absence in the case of a placebo injection. Yawning was clearly described by the patients not as a form discomfort, but as a signal of unblocking, which indicated the beginning of the effect of the relieving treatment [11–14].

Excessive Yawning

The most common cause of frequent and repeated yawning is sleep debt, particularly in children and young adults. Campaigns for the prevention of falling asleep while driving emphasize this warning sign of the risk of falling asleep involuntarily. Research on accident prevention is leading to the development of programs for the automatic detection of yawning and blinking by the driver, in order to trigger an alarm that forces the driver to stop [15]. Drowsiness can be assessed by establishing an Epworth score, in order to uncover a syndrome of sleep apnea or another cause of hypersomnia. In children, drowsiness is often manifested by excessive agitation, punctuated by yawning, with an attention-fixing deficit. Before invoking the diagnosis of a possibly hyperactive child, it is advisable to eliminate any sleep apnea syndrome caused by an obstructive hypertrophy of the tonsils or adenoids. Evans [16] describes, in the same spirit, two cases of inhalation of foreign bodies into the bronchi, which manifested as suffocation alternating with yawning in succession.

Dyspepsia or the sensation of a full stomach and slow digestion, and an irritable colon are often associated with salvos of yawns. Considering the importance of the autonomic nervous system, and the parasympathetic system in particular, in the regulation of digestive functions, it is not surprising that yawning appears to be associated with problems that are essentially functional. The term 'gut brain' or digestive neurology has been used in this context, in order to avoid restricting the pathophysiology of this system to motor deficits, and to also take into account the sensitivity of the digestive system (visceroception, a component of interoception) [17, 18]. The discovery of hypocretin, a neuromediator that triggers sensations of hunger and arousal, could also provide an explanation [19]. It is possible that leptin, the messenger of satiety, and ghrelin, another messenger signaling hunger, play a role that has not yet been elucidated [20]. These functional digestive disorders should be seen in light of a vasovagal episode. The circumstances under which it is triggered are multiple: violent emotion, intense pain, the sight of blood, staying in a confined overheated space, etc. The most common form of the malaise, a loss of consciousness – which occurs in subjects of all ages, regardless of their state of health – is preceded by a rich parade of premonitory disorders that attest to a hyperstimulation of the parasympathetic system: pallor, nausea, salvos of yawning, visual disturbances, etc. The appearance of yawning is a sign that should attract the attention of a health-care worker during invasive exploration, and allow him/her to anticipate a loss of consciousness and subsequent fall. Dorsal decubitus, or an injection of atropine, eliminates the malaise and the yawning [21]. Motion sickness or kinetosis is a related functional disorder that is often accompanied by repetitive yawning before the onset of vomiting [22]. The beginning of hypoglycemia in a diabetic receiving insulin therapy is accompanied by a feeling of hunger, profuse sweating and repeated yawning, similar to the feeling of hunger in non-diabetics.

With a progression that is often insidious, an increase in the frequency of yawning becomes embarrassing both because of the brief pause in activity that it causes, and because of the negative social connotations perceived by both the yawner and the company they are in. Often occurring in salvos of 10–20 successive yawns, the daily number often exceeds 100. Thus, the famous patient presented at the Leçons du Mardi de la Salpêtrière on October 23, 1888 by Prof. J.-M. Charcot [23] yawned 8 times a minute, or 480 times an hour! The most frequent cause, in our times, is of iatrogenic origin. Numerous medications used in neurology and in psychiatry lead to an increase in the frequency of yawning. We will review them here in decreasing order of frequency.

Antidepressants, in particular serotonergic antidepressants, are the ones most often found to be involved [24, 25]. The effect involves the entire pharmacological class, and all molecules studied have been implicated (fluoxetine, paroxetine, escitalopram, duloxetine, venlafaxine, etc.) [26–28]. This symptom is very often wrongly interpreted both by patients and their treatment providers. Attributed to asthenia, the persistence of a depressive state or a lack of effectiveness of the treatment, this frequent repetitive yawning can wrongly lead to an increase in the recommended dosage, which in turn accentuates the problem, whereas stopping the treatment would allow the symptoms to disappear within a few days. There is never any associated somnolence. This effect is sometimes accompanied by erection of the clitoris and involuntary orgasms [29]. Serotonergic antidepressants are nevertheless considered to be better tolerated than tricyclic antidepressants or monoamine oxidase inhibitors. It is not easy to interpret the somewhat inconsistent mechanism controlling this side effect. In fact, in addition to their activity as serotonergic agonists (potentially involving 5-HT_4 receptors), these molecules also have adrenergic, muscarinic cholinergic and histaminergic effects [30, 31]. Unfortunately, as this is only rarely reported to pharmacovigilance agencies, there are no statistics to assess the frequency of this iatrogenic effect, nor any studies showing that it is revealed by association with another psychotropic drug [32]. Curiously, while tricyclic antidepressants have atropinic side effects, thus being inhibitors of yawning, and are reputed to lead to impotence, there have been reports regarding excessively frequent salvos of yawning that accompany involuntary orgasms with clomipramine [33, 34].

Concerning dopamine agonists, we have already discussed apomorphine hydrochloride injected during episodes of motor block in Parkinson's patients in order to restore motor function. It is not possible to invoke a real iatrogenic effect here. Apomorphine hydrochloride, at lower doses administered orally, is used to treat male impotence. Data sheets accompanying the product indicate yawning as a rarely reported side effect seen during the initial clinical studies. Following commercialization, no follow-up data are accessible. Data for other dopaminergic agonists (bromocriptine, lisuride, pergolide, ropinirole, pramipexole, selegiline and piribedil) are no doubt lacking as a result of faulty pharmacovigilance, since animal models show evidence of the same iatrogenic risks [35, 36].

Detoxification after prolonged use in heavy users of coffee or of opiates is accompanied by a withdrawal syndrome that includes the occurrence of repetitive yawning over several days [37–43]. The clinical profile of a neonate with a mother who consumes opiates, legal (methadone, morphine) or not, until the end of her pregnancy, can be striking, with respiratory irregularities and pauses interspersed with salvos of yawning [44, 45].

Migraine is one of the most common disorders in humans, affecting 10–20% of the population at least once per year. It appears to be secondary to a combination of environmental and genetic factors. Clinical and pharmacological findings, as well as recent developments in genetics, confirm the hypothesis that a dysfunction in dopaminergic transmission plays a role in the pathophysiology of a migraine attack. Prodromes (changes in mood, yawning, somnolence, food aversion, etc.) may be related to dopaminergic overstimulation. The dopaminergic system also plays a role in the headache phase, on the one hand by participating in nociceptive pathways, and on the other by intervening in the regulation of cerebral arterial circulation. Apomorphine induces more yawning in migraine sufferers than in non-migraine sufferers [8, 46–48]. The shimmering blind-spot is a classic sign of a visual aura. However, a large number of sufferers have noted that repeated yawning in salvos also acts as an aura before an attack [49–51]. More rarely, the attack ends with repeated yawning, accompanied by drowsiness and a postdrome profile [52, 53].

Yawning can be studied from several angles during the course of a stroke. During the occurrence of an attack (ischemic or hemorrhagic) deficits in vigilance occur, accompanied by salvos of yawning, whether or not the victim is conscious [54–56]. This could be due to intracranial hypertension resulting from the stroke. In the case of a deep coma (Glasgow score = 3), the occurrence of repetitive yawning is a sign of herniation, a grave prognostic sign. Apart from this extremely serious evolution, yawning during the course of a stroke indicates damage to cortical and subcortical circuitry, and to a mechanism of secondary vigilance stimulation controlled by the reticular formation of the brainstem, a mechanism probably common to the yawning that occurs during a partial seizure in temporal lobe epilepsy. During an ischemic attack affecting the territory of the lenticulostriate arteries, damage to the internal capsule and/or the lentiform nucleus leads to complete hemiplegia due to the lesioning of the pyramidal tracts, while the extrapyramidal pathways are spared. In this case, during yawning, the paralyzed arm can be seen to move, bringing the hand up to the mouth. The arm drops immediately following the end of the yawn. We have named this syndrome, which is not a synkinesis, 'parakinesia brachialis oscitans'. With regard to its phylogeny, it has been shown that in quadrupeds like the dog and the horse, there is a synchronization of the ventilatory rhythm with that of gait: one ventilatory cycle per gait cycle, with concomitant acceleration while running. In humans, bipedalism has led to the loss of this automatic synchronization, retaining only the swing of the arms while walking, but no strict synchrony with ventilation. After a stroke has interrupted cortical control, the subjacent neurological structures retrieve their ancestral functions, which are normally inhibited by the overlying cerebral structures as a result of evolution. During the movement of the diaphragm while yawning, the paralyzed arm receives motor stimulation from the lateral reticular nucleus of the medulla, which couples ventilation and locomotion in animals, an extrapyramidal signal that is not inhibited by the ischemic lesion. In two stroke profiles, the persistence of yawning and emotional facial expressions signals the dissociation between automatic and voluntary pathways [57]. In the case of 'locked-in' syndrome caused by an occlusion in the basilar artery territory, there is quadriplegia, in association with bilateral facial paralysis. However, physiological yawning continues to occur [58–60]. Similarly, in bilateral anterior opercular syndrome or Foix-Chavany-Marie syndrome, the muscles of the face, tongue and laryngopharynx are paralyzed during all voluntary acts, including voluntary smiles or grimaces, as well as during language articulation, whereas the expression of emotions, eye blinking, laughing, coughing, swallowing and yawning remain possible. No voluntary imitation of these movements can be carried out. The cause is ischemic, or rarely post-traumatic bilateral damage to the frontoparietal opercular areas [61, 62].

Intracranial hypertension, whether related to a stroke, tumor [63–65] or head trauma [66], can be revealed by headaches and by disturbed vigilance associated with salvos of yawns and with convulsions. Certain coma scores used in the USA take into account the presence of yawning in these situations [67, 68]. Vegetative states of postischemic or other origins also display 'automatic-voluntary dissociation' with the persistence of frequent yawning [69].

J.-M. Charcot presented a patient in 1888, referred to previously, and reported by Gilles de la Tourette [70] in 1890 as suffering from hysteria. Nevertheless, this young woman of 23 years was amenorrheic, epileptic, suffered from a bitemporal loss of the visual field and yawned 480 times an hour. In reality, she was probably developing a prolactinoma of the pituitary gland. I have also personally observed a 39-year-old acromegalic male with prognathism and moderately protruding brows, suffering from persistent asthenia with salvos of almost 200 yawns per day [unpublished data]. Similarly, Wong [65] reported a case of a mucocele of the sphenoid sinus compressing the pituitary stalk, which was revealed by the occurrence of yawning repeated every 15 s. There are a number of clinical arguments to show that an unexplained excess of yawning could be the result of a hypothalamic-pituitary disorder, the mechanism of action of which could be the oversecretion or inappropriate release of oxytocin or other neuromediators due to compression [71, 72].

There has been little interest in the behavioral disturbances that precede or succeed an epileptic seizure by a few minutes to several hours. Nonetheless, these anomalies could provide orienting data that would help to localize the anatomical origin of focal seizures. Before as well as after a temporal, or sometimes a frontal, epileptic seizure, different automatisms such as rubbing the nose with the fingers, yawning or sighing can be observed. J.H. Jackson [73] wrote in around 1876:

> These symptoms do not occur during but after the paroxysm of the seizure; these are movements that are too well coordinated to result from an epileptic discharge; there exists, I think, a double condition: (1) negatively, a loss of control; (2) positively, an augmentation of the activity of the inferior functional center. In any case, the association or the sequence of gestures is very significant.

In accordance with behavioral data, there is a phylogenetic origin to these stereotypical behaviors. They are noticeable during the fetal stage, and continue into the postnatal period and throughout life. Scratching the face, rubbing the nose, yawning and sighing have been described as automatic behaviors that occur before or after absence seizures or focal seizures. They can also be seen in healthy subjects as they awake from sleep. They can be distinguished as being physiological (upon waking) or pathological (for example, in temporal lobe epilepsy) depending on whether their velocity is harmonious or not, and whether their repetition is brief or prolonged. These behavioral automatisms are related to the activation of the brainstem or the spinal cord, the seat of their motor and integrative centers. The cortex, where the seizure is localized, is not involved. Thus, we see the reappearance of ancestral behavioral automatisms that are necessary for survival (such as walking, swimming, mating and other rhythmic activities, to which yawning also belongs), by a liberating ictal cortical disconnection [74–78]. Goldie and Green [79] presented three observations taken from old reports of Gowers [80], Penfield and Jasper [81] and Symonds [82], of children suffering from 'petit mal' seizures, the beginnings of which are signaled by repeated yawning. In addition to the association between temporal lobe epilepsy and yawning, Penfield and Jasper [81] described a rare type of epilepsy, diencephalic epilepsy, the existence of which has been questioned by some epileptologists. It brings together the brutal stimulation of sympathetic and parasympathetic activity: a feeling of disconnection from the environment without loss of consciousness, a 'vasomotor storm' with flush, profuse sweating, rapid rise and fall of the body temperature, pulse and arterial pressure, lacrimation, salivation, pupillary inequality and irregularities of the ventilator rhythm. Salvos of yawning and irrepressible hiccupping accompany this spectacular and very unpleasant profile. The cases described reveal the presence of thalamic tumors [83–87]. D'Mello et al. [88] also reported salvos of yawns as an iatrogenic effect of vibratory massage or of the withdrawal of neuroleptics, persisting several months after convulsions are provoked. He proposed a lesioning of the hypothalamus by way of explanation.

Occurring at the threshold between absence seizures and epilepsy of a psychogenic origin, prolonged hyperventilation (voluntary or unconsciously induced) can alter the level of consciousness, mimicking an epileptic fit, with the appearance of automatic movements such as smiling, swallowing or yawning [89, 90]. Positive or negative emotions are accompanied physiologically by modifications in cardiorespiratory activity, mediated by the autonomic nervous system. Thus, an increase in the frequency of ventilation is one of the signs of a panic attack. The hyperventilation syndrome comprises a neurotic profile on its own, leading to respiratory alkalosis, accompanied in more than 30% of cases by repeated widely spaced yawns that could be seen as a homeostatic counterstimulation of the parasympathetic system [91–95]. The use of relaxation techniques and yoga designed to trigger relaxing yawns allows these problems to be treated [96].

In 2006, in a study published exclusively on the internet, SR Gallezzo of Holyoke Community College (Mass., USA) [97] demonstrated the existence of a link between the frequency of yawning reported by depressive patients and the severity of the depression, using a small sample of 31 patients. Depression was evaluated with the help of the Goldberg scale, and yawning on the basis of a questionnaire proposed by Greco and Baenninger [98]. Statistical analysis of the results demonstrated a significant link: the more the patient yawned, the severer the depressive state. This was the first time that such a study was performed. To the surprise of the author, there was a negative correlation between age and yawning. It should be noted that the number of yawns produced diminishes physiologically with age, and that the predictive value of the relation between yawning and depression is probably lost after 65 years. It should also be remembered that antidepressants, in particularly serotonergic antidepressants, promote repeated yawning.

It is at present quite rare to encounter a schizophrenic who does not take neuroleptics, which, by their mode of action, inhibit yawning. In the past, the reappearance of yawning in a schizophrenic was interpreted as a resumption of contact with the environment and socialization [99]. Salvos of yawns, such as those seen in at least three of the five cases reported by Gilles de la Tourette in 1890, could have a psychogenic cause, as a form of non-verbal language. These have been described as an urgent and irrepressible feeling, following a sensation of epigastric heaviness with ascendant retrosternal constriction, relieved by undergoing a ventilatory period of yawning that yields a brief feeling of pleasure such as those described by patients affected by nervous tics [100, 101].

Sandy [102] reported a series of 5 patients in the initial stages of Steele-Richardson-Olszewski syndrome, or progressive supranuclear palsy, with balance deficits, oculomotor problems and salvos of repeated yawning that were reduced, paradoxically, by the administration of dopaminergic agonists. Louwerse [103] reported, in a series of 200 patients with the bulbar form of amyotrophic lateral sclerosis or Charcot's disease, the existence of excessive yawning in salvos in around 10% of them, which is also the case in the study carried out by Williams [104]. Wicks [105] saw this problem in 47% of patients (n = 539). Present during the initial phase of the disease and concurrent with the appearance of swallowing deficits, the yawning disappears with the aggravation of paralysis. A brainstem attack in multiple sclerosis can yield the same profile [106].

Between 1917 and 1925, an epidemic of encephalitis described as lethargic by C. von Economo (1876–1931) [107] struck the whole of Europe. After an initial meningitic phase, a lethargic phase lasting several weeks set in. These acute symptoms, often fatal, were followed in those who survived by a 'chaos of abnormal movements' (Pierre Marie), with the mixing of depressive or delirious manifestations, oculogyric crises, Parkinsonian syndromes, etc. In 1921, Sicard and Paraff [108] reported observations in which the initial lethargic phase was followed by spasmodic attacks of hiccupping, laughing or crying, and salvos of repetitive yawning several times a day. The homogeneity of the process of morbidity and the relative consistency of the lesion sites were in contrast to the polymorphism of the clinical manifestations. Contemporary discoveries confirm the soundness of the hypotheses put forward by C. von Economo. Autoimmune injury to the basal ganglia of the hypothalamus leads to a rarefaction of orexin/hypocretin-containing neurons, among others, and decreases, either transiently or permanently, the secretion of certain neuromediators responsible for arousal.

Yawning Triggers a Disorder

The act of yawning is not merely a simple opening of the mouth but a complex coordinated movement, bringing together a flexion followed by an extension of the neck, a wide dilatation of the laryngopharynx with maximal descent, and an opening of the eustachian tubes [109]. Each of these elements can lead to pain or to dysfunctions.

Yawning is the most frequent cause of mandibular subluxation, ahead of laughing, vomiting and dental care. The subluxation is anterior; in other words, the mandibular condyle juts out in front of the temporal condyle and into the temporal fossa, from which it cannot be extricated due to the tonicity of the masticator muscles. The subluxation is most often bilateral. It is generally possible to reduce it promptly without anesthesia [110, 111]. Relapses occur frequently. Although this type of luxation may occur during normal physiological yawning [112–115], several publications have described mandibular luxation as a complication of uncontrollable yawning while on serotonergic antidepressants [116, 117] or during the induction of anesthesia [118–120].

In addition, yawning can trigger painful cramps in the geniohyoid muscle [121].

When a patient presents with otalgia (showing no noticeable lesion of the ear) or for atypical facial pain, the presence of pain aggravated by yawning is a good indication of a disorder of the temporomandibular joints, such as arthritis, ankylosis, mandibular dysfunctions or myalgias of the masticator muscles [122–125].

Yawning can be the release mechanism or the trigger for an attack of glossopharyngeal neuralgia [126, 127]. As in the case of swallowing, it can initiate choreoathetotic movements of the lips and the laryngopharynx, following a brainstem stroke [128]. In 2001, D.E. Jacome described two patients with paroxysmal headaches, in whom the only triggering factor was yawning [129, 130]. In 2004, he described two other cases in which yawning led to extracephalic pain that appeared neuralgic [131]. In the first case, neck pain radiated towards a shoulder, and in the second, intense pain invaded the anterior portion of the neck, where a thyroid tumor of the clear-cell carcinoma type was developing. In both cases, a spontaneous wide opening of the mouth did not trigger pain; this was only triggered by yawning. Another clinical type of neuralgia that can be triggered by yawning is short-lasting neuralgiform unilateral pain affecting the orbital-periorbital area and associated with autonomic phenomena consisting mainly of conjunctival injection, tearing, and rhinorrhea (Charlin-Sluder syndrome) [132].

The Marin Amat syndrome (or inverted Marcus Gunn syndrome) consists of a synkinetic closing of the eyelids of one eye while opening the mouth, notably during yawning [133].

Fractures of a long styloid apophysis are rare. Throat or neck pain, reduced neck mobility, hoarseness and a lateral mass in the neck are all signs that point to this condition. They occur secondary to yawning or a direct shock, such as those encountered during a traffic accident [134, 135]. These should prompt a search for an Eagle's syndrome – in which lateral neck pain, triggered by yawning or mastication, is associated with the pressure exerted by the styloid process within the tonsillar fossa [136, 137]. X-rays of the neck reveal the calcification of the stylohyoid ligaments (a discovery that sometimes occurs by chance), which becomes symptomatic whether or not there is a fracture [138, 139].

Idiopathic carotidynia is a controversial diagnosis, based on clinical arguments. The international classification of headache disorders established by the International Headache Society proposes the presence of at least one of the following criteria in order to retain this diagnosis: localized hypersensitivity, swelling and an increase in pulsations. The pain is typically unbearable, pulsatile, permanent and localized at the carotid bifurcation, but it may radiate towards the mandible, cheek, eye or ear. The symptoms are often exacerbated by swallowing, chewing, yawning and contralateral movements of the neck. The cardinal clinical sign is an exaggerated sensitivity of the carotid bulb to palpation, which often reveals prominent swelling with an accentuation of visible and palpable pulsations. Other serious causes (dissection of the carotid) should be excluded. Its evolution appears to be benign in most cases [140, 141].

Yawning Relieves a Disorder

The eustachian tubes play a role in the aeration of the middle ear, or pressure equalization [142]. Physiologically, the eustachian tubes open during swallowing due to the contraction of the peristaphyline muscles. Defective opening occurs as a result of tube dysfunctions. These could be a consequence of inflammatory phenomena affecting the ear and throat, or functional phenomena, such as during variations in pressure during air travel. The powerful contraction of the peristaphyline muscles during yawning explains its airing effect on the tympanic cavity, which serves to restore hearing in case of serous otitis or during rapid descent while in flight [143, 144].

Dysbaric facial paralysis is a rare event, but one which usually has a favorable outcome. It is linked to a change in pressure in the medium in which the victim evolves, and is responsible for ischemic neuropraxia of the facial nerve, e.g. during diving or flying. If hyperbaric oxygen therapy is not available immediately, either the Toynbee maneuver, provoked yawning or swallowing can accelerate recovery and limit the risk of sequelae [145].

The extrinsic or intrinsic musculature of the larynx is particularly sensitive to emotional stress. Its hypercontraction is a common denominator in all forms of functional or psychogenic dysphonia and aphonia. Yawning-whistling is a technique that has come into increasing use over the last few years, in particular as a therapy for vocal fatigue. The technique is particularly effective in combating the excessive elevation of the larynx and constriction of the glottis that characterize vocal fatigue. This condition corresponds to an excessive muscular effort by the respiratory, vocal and resonance systems, which tends to raise the larynx. This technique aims to open the glottis and to reposition the larynx at its lowest point in order to reduce muscular effort to a minimum, which is what yawning accomplishes physiologically.

Pieter Brueghel the Elder painted, in around 1560, a work posthumously named *The Yawner*, currently on display at the Royal Museums of Fine Arts in Brussels. Marsden [146] contests this interpretation and believes that it depicts a blepharospasm or oromandibular dystonia, the contraction of which can be relieved by yawning, as noted by a good number of patients.

Concluding Remarks

At the end of this vast panorama, the consultation of a patient complaining of excessive yawning can be schematized. The first step consists of looking for an iatrogenic effect, the most frequent cause. Then, a search for abnormal drowsiness or sleep debt should allow any syndrome of sleep apnea to be uncovered. Functional causes leading to an anxiety disorder, possibly associated with a hyperventilation syndrome, should be treated by relaxation and yoga. This should be correlated with the occurrence of dyspepsia. Clinical examination is needed to detect pituitary/hypophyseal endocrine anomalies, intracranial hypertensive syndromes, partial temporal seizure, stroke or Charcot's disease. Finally, repeated yawning could form part of a tic disease.

References

1 Meige H, Feindel G: Les tics et leur traitement. Paris, Masson, 1902, p 633.
2 Craig AD: Interoception: the sense of the physiological condition of the body. Curr Opin Neurobiol 2003;13:500–505.
3 Craig AD: How do you feel – now? The anterior insula and human awareness. Nature Rev Neurosci 2009;10:59–70.
4 Mogilnicka E, Klimek V: Drugs affecting dopamine neurons and yawning behavior. Pharmacol Biochem Behav 1977;7:303–305.
5 Colosimo C, Pontieri FE: Yawning in Parkinson's disease. Neurology 1999;52:428.
6 Collins GT, Newman AH, Grundt P, et al: Yawning and hypothermia in rats: effects of dopamine D_3 and D_2 agonists and antagonists. Psychopharmacology (Berl) 2007;193:159–170.
7 Blin O, Masson G, Azulay JP, Fondarai J, Serratrice G: Apomorphine-induced blinking and yawning in healthy volunteers. Br J Clin Pharmacol 1990;30: 769–773.

8 Blin O, Azulay JP, Masson G, Aubrespy G, et al: Apomorphine-induced yawning in migraine patients: enhanced responsiveness. Clin Neuropharmacol 1991;14:91–95.
9 Goren J, Friedman J: Yawning: an aura for an L-DOPA induced 'on' in Parkinson's disease. Neurology 1998;50:823.
10 Dewey RB, Hutton JT, Lewitt PA, Factor SA: A randomized, double-blind, placebo-controlled trial of subcutaneously injected apomorphine for parkinsonian of state events. Arch Neurol 2001;58:1385–1392.
11 Kolls BJ, Stacy M: Apomorphine: a rapid rescue agent for the management of motor fluctuations in advanced Parkinson disease. Clin Neuropharmacol 2006;29:292–301.
12 Lal S: Apomorphine in the evaluation of dopaminergic function in man. Progr Neuropsychopharmacol Biol Psychol 1988;12:117–164.
13 Lal S, Tesfaye Y, Thavundayil JX, et al: Effect of time-of-day on yawning response to apomorphine in normal subjects. Neuropsychobiology 2000;44: 178–180.
14 Lewitt PA, Ondo WG, Van Lunen B, et al: Open-label study assessment of safety and adverse effects of subcutaneous apomorphine injections in treating 'off' episodes in advanced Parkinson disease. Clin Neuropharmacol 2009;32:89–93.
15 Benoit A, Caplier A: Hypovigilence analysis: open or closed eye or mouth? Blinking or yawning frequency? Advanced Video and Signal Based Surveillance 2005:207–212.
16 Evans EB: Yawning in pharyngeal obstruction. Br Med J1978;1:443–444.
17 Cameron OG: Visceral Sensory Neuroscience: Interoception. Oxford, Oxford University Press, 2002.
18 Grover M, Drossman DA: Psychopharmacologic and behavioral treatments for functional gastrointestinal disorders. Gastrointest Endosc Clin N Am 2009;19:151–170.
19 Sato-Suzuki I, Kita I, Seki Y, et al: Cortical arousal induced by microinjection of orexins into the paraventricular nucleus of the rat. Behav Brain Res 2002; 128:169–177.
20 Adamantidis A, de Lecea L: Sleep and metabolism: shared circuits, new connections. Trends Endocrinol Metab 2008;19:362–370.
21 Cronin TG: Yawning: an early manifestation of vasovagal reflex. Am J Roentgenol 1988;150:209.
22 Graybiel A, Knepton J: Sopite syndrome: a sometimes sole manifestation of motion sickness. Aviat Space Environ Med 1976;47:873–882.
23 Charcot JM: Leçons du mardi à La Salpêtrière. Paris, Lecrosnier & Babé, 1889.
24 Beale MD, Murphree TM: Excessive yawning and SSRI therapy. Int J Neuropsycho Pharmacol 2000; 3:275–276.
25 Gutierrez-Alvarez AM: Do your patients suffer from excessive yawning? Acta Psychiat Scandinavica 2007;115:80–81.
26 Chen CH, Lu ML: Venlafaxine-induced excessive yawning. Prog Neuropsychopharmacol Biol Psychiatry 2009;33:156–157.
27 De Las Cuevas C, Sanz EJ: Duloxetine-induced excessive disturbing and disabling yawning. J Clin Psychopharmacol 2007;27:106–107.
28 Harada KI: Paroxetine-induced excessive yawning. Psychiat Clin Neurosci 2006;60:260.
29 Modell JG: Repeated observations of yawning, clitoral engorgement, and orgasm associated with fluoxetine administration. J Clin Psychopharmacol 1989; 9:63–65.
30 Cooper SJ, Dourish CT: Neural basis of drug induced yawning; in Cooper SJ, Dourish CT (ed): Neurobiology of Stereotyped Behaviour. Oxford, Clarendon Press, 1990, pp 91–116.
31 Urba-Holmgren R, Holmgren B, Rodriguez R, et al: Serotoninergic modulation of yawning. Pharmacol Biochem Behav 1979;11:371–372.
32 Sommet A, Desplas M, Lapeyre-Mestre M, Montastruc JL: Drug-induced yawning: a review of the French pharmacovigilance database. Drug Saf 2007;30:327–331.
33 Goldberg RL: Sustained yawning as a side effect of imipramine. Int J Psychiatry Med 1983;13:277–280.
34 McLean JD, Forsythe RG, Kapkin IA: Unusual side effects of clomipramine associated with yawning. Can J Psychiatry 1983;28:569–570.
35 Furukawa T: Yawning behavior for preclinical drug evaluation. Meth Find Exp Clin Phamacol 1996;18: 141–155.
36 Mogilnicka E, Klimek V: Drugs affecting dopamine neurons and yawning behavior. Pharmacol Biochem Behav 1977;7:303–305.
37 Evans SM, Griffiths RR: Caffeine withdrawal: a parametric analysis of caffeine dosing conditions. J Pharmacol Exp Ther 1999;289:285–294.
38 Freye E, Levy J: Acute abstinence syndrome following abrupt cessation of long-term use of tramadol: a case study. Eur J Pain 2000;4:307–311.
39 Freye E, Levy J: Constitutive opioid receptor activation: a prerequisite mechanism involved in acute opioid withdrawal. Addict Biol 2005;10:131–137.
40 Gowing L, Ali R, White J: Buprenorphine for the management of opioid withdrawal. Cochrane Database Syst Rev 2004;(4):CDO2025.

41 Hiltunen AJ, Lafolie P, Martel J, Ottosson EC, Boreus LO, Beck O, Borg S, Hjemdahl P: Subjective and objective symptoms in relation to plasma methadone concentration in methadone patients. Psychopharmacology (Berl) 1995;118:122–126.
42 Lane JD, Phillips-Bute BG: Caffeine deprivation affects vigilance performance and mood. Physiol Behav 1998;65:171–175.
43 Phillips-Bute BG, Lane JD: Caffeine withdrawal symptoms following brief caffeine deprivation Physiol Behav 1997;63:35–39.
44 Ostrea EM Jr, Chavez CJ, Strauss ME: A study of factors that influence the severity of neonatal narcotic withdrawal. Addict Dis 1975;2:187–199.
45 Robe LB, Gromisch DS, Iosub S: Symptoms of neonatal ethanol withdrawal. Curr Alcohol 1981;8:485–493.
46 Blau JN: Migraine postdromes: symptoms after attacks. Cephalalgia 1991;11:229–231.
47 Cerbo R, Barbanti P, Buzzi MG, et al: Dopamine hypersensitivity in migraine: role of the apomorphine test. Clin Neuropharmacol 1997;20:36–44.
48 Del Bene E, Poggioni M: Video assessment of yawning induced by sublingual apomorphine in migraine. Headache 1994;34:536–538.
49 Jacome DE: Compulsive yawning as migraine premonitory symptom. Cephalalgia 2001;21:623–625.
50 Jacome DE: Primary yawning headache. Cephalalgia 2001;2:697–699.
51 Quintela E, Castillo J, Munoz P, et al: Premonitory and resolution symptoms in migraine: a prospective study in 100 unselected patients. Cephalalgia 2006;26:1051–1060.
52 Blau JN, Engel HO: Premonitory and prodromal symptoms in cluster headache. Cephalalgia 1998;18:91–93.
53 Schoonman GG, Evers DJ, Terwindt GM, et al: The prevalence of premonitory symptoms in migraine: a questionnaire study in 461 patients. Cephalalgia 2006;26:1209–1213.
54 Cattaneo L, Cucurachi L, Chierici E, et al: Pathological yawning as a presenting symptom of brainstem ischaemia in two patients. JNNP 2006;77:98–100.
55 Singer OC, Humpich MC, Lanfermann H, Neumann-Haefelin T: Yawning in acute anterior circulation stroke. J Neurol Neurosurg Psychiatry 2007;78:1253–1254.
56 Walusinski O: Yawning and stroke (editorial commentaries). J Neurol Neurosurgery Psychiatry 2007;78:1166.
57 Walusinski O, Bogousslavsky J, Neau JP: Hand up! Yawn and raise your arm. Int J Stroke 2010;5:21–27.
58 Bauer G, Gerstenbrand F, Hengl W: Involuntary motor phenomena in the locked-in syndrome. J Neurol 1980;223:191–198.
59 Bauer G, Prugger M, Rumpl E: Stimulus evoked oral automatisms in the locked-in syndrome. Arch Neurol 1982;39:435–436.
60 Krasnianski M, Gaul C, Neudecker S, et al: Yawning despite trismus in a patient with locked-in syndrome caused by a thrombosed megadolichobasilar artery. Clin Neurol Neurosurg 2003;106:44–46.
61 Billeth R, Jorgler E, Baumhackl U: Bilateral anterior operculum syndrome. Nervenarzt 2000;71:651–654.
62 Laurent-Vannier A, Fadda G, Laigle P, et al: Syndrome de Foix Chavany Marie d'origine traumtaique. Rev Neurol 1999;155:387–390.
63 Arai K, Kita K, Komiyama A, et al: Progressive dysautonomia in hemangioblastoma in the region of the fourth ventricle. No To Shinkei 1986;38:195–200.
64 Gschwend J: Yawning in a case with transsecting glioma of the pons (in German). Fortschr Neurol Psychiatr Grenzgeb 1977;45:652–655.
65 Wong KY, Ngan KC, Sin VC, et al: Sphenoidal sinus mucocoele and yawning after radiation treatment for nasopharyngeal carcinoma. Clinical Oncol 1997;9:415–417.
66 Jurko MF, Andy OJ: Post-lesion yawning and thalamotomy site. Appl Neurophysiol 1975;38:73–79.
67 Crosby L, Parsons LC: Clinical neurologic assessment tool: development and testing of an instrument to index neurologic status. Heart Lung 1989;18:121–129.
68 Bateman DE: Neurological assessment of coma. J Neurol Neurosurg Psychiatry 2001;71:113–117.
69 Manish M, Veenu S: Persistent vegetative state. Neurology 2007;68:1635.
70 Gilles de la Tourette G, Huet E, Guinon G: Contribution à l'étude des bâillements hystériques: Nouvelle Iconographie de la Salpêtrière. Paris, Lecrosnier & Babé, 1890, pp 97–119.
71 de Wied D: Behavioral pharmacology of neuropeptides related to melanocortins and the neurohypophyseal hormones. Eur J Pharmacol 1999;375:1–11.
72 Sato F, Aoki H, Nakamura K, et al: Suppressive effects of chronic hyperprolactinemia on penile erection and yawning following administration of apomorphine to pituitary-transplanted rats. J Androl 1997;18:21–25.
73 Jackson JH: Selected Writings of John Hughlings Jackson Edited by James Taylor: On Epilepsy and Epileptiform Convulsions. London, Basic Books, 1931.

74 Medrano V, Selles-Galiana MF, Fernandez-Izquierdo S, et al: Yawning and temporal lobe epilepsy. Rev Neurol (Spain) 2005;4:63–64.

75 Muchnik S, Finkielman S, Semeniuk G, de Aguirre MI: Yawning and temporal lobe epilepsy. Medicina (B Aires) 2003;63:137–139.

76 Muchnik S, Finkielman S, Semeniuk G, de Aguirre MI: Yawning. Medicina (B Aires) 2003;63:229–232.

77 Tassinari CA, Gardella E, Meletti S, et al: The neuro-ethological interpretation of motor behaviours in 'nocturnal-hyperkinetic-frontalseizures': emergence of 'innate' motor behaviours and role of central pattern generators; in Beaumanoir A, Andermann F, Chauvel P, et al: Frontal Seizures and Epilepsies in Children. Montrouge, J. Libbey Eurotext, 2003, pp 43–48.

78 Yankovsky AE, Andermann F, Dubeau F: Post-ictal forceful yawning in a patient with nondominant hemisphere epilepsy. Epileptic Disord 2006;8:65–69.

79 Goldie L, Green JM: Yawning and epilepsy. J Psychosom Res 1961;5:263–268.

80 Gowers WR: Epilepsy and other chronic convulsive diseases: their causes, symptoms & treatment. New York, William Wood, 1885.

81 Penfield W, Jasper H: Epilepsy and the functional anatomy of the human brain. Boston, Little, Brown & Company, 1954.

82 Symonds CP: Discussion on faints and fits. Proc Royal Soc Med 1950;43:507–518.

83 Andy OJ, Jurko M: Diencephalic seizures. Appl Neurophysiol 1983;46:62–67.

84 Boeve BF, Wijdicks EF, Benarroch EE, et al: Paroxysmal sympathetic storms ('diencephalic seizures') after severe diffuse axonal head injury. Mayo Clin Proc 1998;73:148–152.

85 Bullard DE: Diencephalic seizures: responsiveness to bromocriptine and morphine. Ann Neurol 1987;21:609–611.

86 Giroud M, Sautreaux JL, Thierry A, et al: Diencephalic epilepsy with congenital suprasellar arachnoid cyst in an infant. Childs Nerv Syst 1988;4:252–254.

87 Goh KY, Conway EJ, Da Rosso RC, et al: Sympathetic storms in a child with a midbrain glioma: a variant of diencephalic seizures. Pediatr Neurol 1999;21:742–744.

88 D'Mello DA, Vincent FM, Lerner MP: Yawning as a complication of electroconvulsive therapy and concurrent neuroleptic withdrawal. J Nerv Ment Dis 1988;176:188–189.

89 Lum LM, Connolly MB, Farrell K, et al: Hyperventilation-induced high-amplitude rhythmic slowing with altered awareness: a video-EEG comparison with absence seizures. Epilepsia 2002;43:1372–1378.

90 Lafleur J, Reiher J: Pseudo-absences. EEG Clin Neurophysiol 1977;43:279–280.

91 Bidat E, Sznajder M, Fermanian C, et al: A diagnostic questionnaire for the hyperventilation syndrome in children. Rev Mal Respir 2008;25:829–838.

92 Klein DF: False suffocation alarms, spontaneous panics, and related conditions, an integrative hypothesis. Arch Gen Psychiatry 1993;50:306–317.

93 Nardi AE, Freire RC, Zin WA: Panic disorder and control of breathing. Respir Physiol Neurobiol 2009;167:133–143.

94 Philippot P, Chapelle G, Blairy S: Respiratory feedback in the generation of emotion. Cogn Emot 2002;16:605–627.

95 Saper CB: The central autonomic nervous system: conscious visceral perception and autonomic pattern generation. Annu Rev Neurosci 2002;25:433–469.

96 Brown RP, Gerbarg PL: Sudarshan Kriya yogic breathing in the treatment of stress, anxiety and depression. J Alternat Complement Med 2005;11:189–201.

97 Gallezzo SR: Examining the connection between yawning and depression. 2006. http://baillement.com/recherche/gallezzo.html.

98 Greco M, Baenninger R: On the context of yawning: when, where and why? Psychol Rec 1993;43:175–183.

99 Beckmann H, Zimmer R: An ethological interpretation of stereotypy induced by environmental stimulus. Arch Psychiatr Nervenkr 1981;230:81–89.

100 Marcus N: Yawning: analytic and therapeutic considerations. Int J Child Psychotherapy 1973;2:406–418.

101 Shilkret H: Psychogenic sneezing and yawning. Psychosom Med 1949;11:127–128.

102 Sandyk R: Excessive yawning and progressive supranuclear palsy. Int J Neurosci 1987;34:123–124.

103 Louwerse E: Forced yawning as a pseudo-bulbar sign in amyotrophic lateral sclerosis. J Neurosci Sci 1998;54(suppl):332.

104 Williams DR: The yawning reflex: an upper motor neuron sign in amyotrophic lateral sclerosis. Neurology 2000;55:1592–1593.

105 Wicks P: Excessive yawning is common in the bulbar-onset form of ALS. Acta Psychiatr Scand 2007;116:76.

106 Postert T, Pöhlau D, Meves S, et al: Pathological yawning as a symptom of multiple sclerosis. J Neurol 1996;243:300–301.

107 von Economo C: Encephalitis Lethargica: Its Sequellae and Treatment. London, Oxford University Press, 1931.
108 Sicard JA, Paraff A: Fou rire syncopal et bâillements au cours de l'encéphalite épidémique. Bull Mém Soc Méd Hôp Paris 1921;45:232.
109 Zafar H, Nordh E, Eriksson PO: Temporal coordination between mandibular and head-neck movements during jaw opening-closing tasks in man. Arch Oral Biol 2000;45:675–682.
110 Chan TC, Harrigan RA, Ufberg J, et al: Mandibular reduction. J Emerg Med 2008;34:435–440.
111 Gugle MM: Etiology, pathogenesis and treatment of habitual dislocations of the T.M. Joints. Indian J Dent Res 2002;13:88–94.
112 Forté MC: Le Bâillement; thesis, 1982, n°117, Amicale Corporative des Etudiants en Médecine de Bordeaux, p 89.
113 Myrhaug H: Luxation of the mandible in yawning. Tidsskr Nor Laegeforen 1961;81:362–365.
114 Ndiokwelu E: Bilateral dislocation of the mandible: 2 cases in a nuclear family. Odontostomatol Trop 2005;28:27–30.
115 Ugboko VI, Oginni FO, Ajike SO, et al: A survey of temporomandibular joint dislocation: aetiology, demographics, risk factors and management in 96 Nigerian cases. Int J Oral Maxillofac Surg 2005;34: 499–502.
116 Tesfaye Y, Lal S: Hazard of yawning. CMAJ 1990; 142:15.
117 Pae CU, Kim JJ, Lee CU, Lee SJ, et al: Injured temporomandibular joint associated with fluoxetine-monotherapy-induced repeated yawning. Gen Hosp Psychiatry 2003;25:217–218.
118 Avidan A: Dislocation of the temporomandibular joint due to forceful yawning during induction with propofol. J Clin Anesth 2002;14:159–160.
119 Quessard A, Barrière P, Levy F, et al: Delayed diagnosis of a postanaesthesia temporomandibular joint dislocation. Ann Fr Anesth Reanim 2008;27:846–849.
120 Unnikrishnan KP, Sinha PK, Rao S: Mandibular dislocation from yawning during induction of anesthesia. Can J Anaesth 2006;53:1164–1165.
121 André-Thomas, de Ajuriaguerra J: Etude sémiologique du tonus musculaire. Paris, Flammarion, 1949, p 844.
122 Helöe B, Helöe LA: Frequency and distribution of myofascial pain-dysfunction syndrome in a population of 25-year-olds. Community Dent Oral Epidemiol 1979;7:357–360.
123 Marcos MM, Velicia MR, Aguirre JJ: Primary stabbing headache with buccal triggers. Eur Neurol 2005;53:91–92.
124 Nassif NJ, Talic YF: Classic symptoms in temporomandibular disorder patients: a comparative study. Cranio 2001;19:33–34.
125 Yap AU, Chua EK, Hoe JK: Clinical TMD: pain-related disability and psychological status of TMD patients. J Oral Rehabil 2002;29:374–378.
126 Minagar A, Sheremata W: Glossopharyngeal neuralgia and multiple sclerosis. Neurology 2000;54: 1368–1370.
127 Skelton A, Fried R: Headphone neuralgia. N Engl J Med 1995;333:1786–1787.
128 Riley DE: Paroxysmal kinesigenic dystonia associated with a medullary lesion. Mov Disord 1996;11: 738–740.
129 Jacome DE: Compulsive yawning as migraine premonitory symptom. Cephalalgia 2001;2:623–625.
130 Jacome DE: Primary yawning headache. Cephalalgia 2001;21:697–699.
131 Jacome DE: Extracephalic yawning pain. Cephalalgia 2004;24:411–413.
132 Lagares A, Gomez P, Perez-Nunez A, et al: Short-lasting unilateral neuralgiform headache with conjunctival injection and tearing syndrome. Neurosurgery 2005;56:E413.
133 Oh JY, Kim JE, Park KD, et al: A case of familial inverse Marcus Gunn phenomenon. J Neurol Neurosurg Psychiatry 2003;74:277–282.
134 McGinnis JM Jr: Fracture of an ossified stylohyoid bone. Arch Otolaryngol 1981;107:460.
135 McCorkell SJ: Fractures of the styloid process and stylohyoid ligament: an uncommon injury. J Trauma 1985;25:1010–1012.
136 Feldman VB: Eagle's syndrome: a case of symptomatic calcification of the stylohyoid ligaments. J Can Chiropr Assoc 2003;47:21–27.
137 Klécha A, Hafian H, Devauchelle B, et al: A report of post-traumatic Eagle's syndrome. Int J Oral Maxillofac Surg 2008;37:970–997.
138 Fanibunda K, Lovelock DJ: Calcified styloid ligament: unusual pressure symptoms. Dentomaxillofacial Radiol 1997;26:249–251.
139 Mupparapu M, Robinson MD: The mineralized and elongated styloid process: a review of current diagnostic criteria and evaluation strategies. Gen Dent 2005;53:54–59.
140 O'Neill B, Aronson A, Pearson B, Nauss L: Superior laryngeal neuralgia: carotidynia or just another pain in the neck? Headache1982;22:6–9.
141 Hill LM, Hastings G: Carotidynia: a pain syndrome. J Fam Pract 1994;39:71–75.
142 Winther B, Gwaltney JM Jr, Phillips CD, et al: Radiopaque contrast dye in nasopharynx reaches the middle ear during swallowing and/or yawning. Acta Otolaryngol 2005;125:625–628.

143 Laskiewicz A: Yawning with regard to the respiratory organs and the ear. Acta Oto laryngologica (Stockholm) 1953;43:267–270.
144 Lepp FH: Remarques sur la signification physiologique du bâillement. Bull Group Int Rech Sci Stomtol Odontol 1982;25:251–290.
145 d'Andréa C, Méliet JL, Staikowski F: Peripheral facial palsy secondary to middle-ear overpressure. Presse Med 2008;37:643–647.
146 Marsden CD: Blepharospasm-oromandibular dystonia syndrome. J Neurol Neurosurg Psychiatry 1976; 39:1204–1209.

Dr. Olivier Walusinski
20 rue de Chartres
FR–28160 Brou (France)
Tel. +33 2 37 47 07 77, Fax +33 2 37 47 19 07
E-Mail walusinski@baillement.com

Author Index

Subject Index